the**facts**

Psoriatic arthritis

D1638567

also available in thefacts series

the**facts**

Psoriatic arthritis

Dafna D. Gladman MD, FRCPC

Professor of Medicine, University of Toronto;
Senior Scientist, Toronto Western Research Institute;
University Health Network, Toronto Western Hospital,
Toronto, Ontario, Canada

Vinod Chandran MBBS, MD, DM

Clinical Research Fellow, University of Toronto;
Centre for Prognosis Studies in the Rheumatic Diseases;
University Health Network, Toronto Western Hospital,
Toronto, Ontario, Canada

OXFORD
UNIVERSITY PRESS

OXFORD
UNIVERSITY PRESS

Great Clarendon Street, Oxford OX2 6DP

Oxford University Press is a department of the University of Oxford.
It furthers the University's objective of excellence in research, scholarship,
and education by publishing worldwide in

Oxford New York

Auckland Cape Town Dar es Salaam Hong Kong Karachi
Kuala Lumpur Madrid Melbourne Mexico City Nairobi
New Delhi Shanghai Taipei Toronto

With offices in

Argentina Austria Brazil Chile Czech Republic France Greece
Guatemala Hungary Italy Japan Poland Portugal Singapore
South Korea Switzerland Thailand Turkey Ukraine Vietnam

Oxford is a registered trade mark of Oxford University Press
in the UK and in certain other countries

Published in the United States
by Oxford University Press Inc., New York

British Library Cataloguing in Publication Data
Data available

Library of Congress Cataloguing in Publication Data
Data available

Typeset in Plantin
by Cepha Imaging Pvt. Ltd., Bangalore, India
Printed in China
on acid-free paper by
Asia Pacific Offset

ISBN 978–0–19–923122–5 (Pbk.)

1 3 5 7 9 10 8 6 4 2

Contents

1

What is psoriatic arthritis?

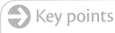

> ## Key points
>
> - Psoriasis is a chronic inflammatory skin condition
>
> - Psoriatic arthritis is an inflammatory arthritis occurring in patients with psoriasis
>
> - Psoriatic arthritis affects 10–30% of patients with psoriasis
>
> - Psoriatic arthritis affects the peripheral and spinal joints
>
> - CASPAR criteria facilitate the diagnosis

Psoriasis is a chronic inflammatory skin condition which presents most commonly with red plaques over the extensor surfaces of the elbows and knees, as well as in the scalp (Fig. 1.1, p. 2). Specific nail lesions are also common in patients with psoriasis (Fig. 1.2).

Historical perspective

The occurrence of a form of arthritis among patients with psoriasis was first noted in the nineteenth century, although evidence of the disease was noted in archeological findings from the Judean desert, dating the disease much earlier than that. Baron Aliberti first described the association between psoriasis and arthritis (Table 1.1). Later in the nineteenth century several French physicians recognized the presence of a form of arthritis among patients with psoriasis. However, over the ensuing years many investigators considered the arthritis associated with psoriasis to be a variant of rheumatoid arthritis, which was the main known inflammatory form of arthritis at the time. Psoriatic arthritis was finally recognized as an entity separate from rheumatoid arthritis

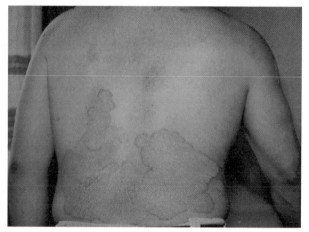

Figure 1.1 Lesions typical of chronic plaque psoriasis on the back.

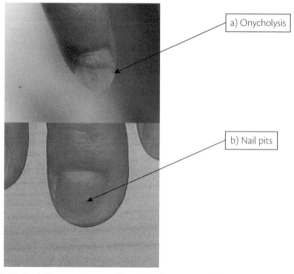

a) Onycholysis

b) Nail pits

Figure 1.2 Typical changes seen on the nails of patients with psoriasis.

when it was found that the majority of patients with psoriatic arthritis were negative for a test for **rheumatoid factor**. Rheumatoid factor is a test discovered in 1948 that is found to be positive in about 85% of patients with rheumatoid arthritis but in fewer than 15% of patients with psoriatic arthritis. Patients who are negative for rheumatoid factor are said to be '**seronegative**'.

 Myth

Psoriatic arthritis is the chance occurrence of inflammatory arthritis in patients with psoriasis.

 Fact

Psoriatic arthritis is a specific inflammatory arthritis that occurs commonly in patients with psoriasis.

Thus, it was only in the latter half of the twentieth century, with the classical descriptions of the varied presentations of psoriatic arthritis by Professor Verna Wright and Dr John Moll in Leeds, UK, that psoriatic arthritis truly

Table 1.1 History of psoriatic arthritis

1818	Baron Jean Luis Aliberti describes association between psoriasis and arthritis
1860	Pierre Bazin uses term 'psoriasis arthritique'
1888	Charles Bourdillon writes a doctoral thesis entitled 'Psoriasis et Arthropathies'
1937	Jeghers and Robinson hold that psoriatic arthritis is a unique entity
1939	Bauer writes: 'there is little justification for considering these patients as suffering from a distinct disease entity'
1951	Vilanova and Pinol describe psoriatic arthritis
1956	Wright reports on psoriasis and arthritis
1958	Cost and colleagues report on a large series of psoriatic arthritis patients
1959	Wright compares psoriatic arthritis and rheumatoid arthritis
1964	The American Rheumatism Association (ARA) recognizes psoriatic arthritis as an entity

became an accepted entity in itself. Psoriatic arthritis was defined by Moll and Wright as an inflammatory arthritis associated with psoriasis, usually seronegative for rheumatoid factor. Finally, in 1964 psoriatic arthritis received a unique recognition by the American College of Rheumatology.

Epidemiological evidence

There is very good evidence that the incidence of arthritis in the presence of psoriasis is increased above what would normally be expected in the population (Fig. 1.3). Whereas in the general population the prevalence of inflammatory arthritis is 3–5%, among patients with psoriasis this frequency is increased to 10–30%. Moreover, the frequency of psoriasis in the general population is estimated at 2–3%, while among patients with arthritis the frequency of psoriasis is at least 7%. A recent study from France suggests that as many as 18% of patients with arthritis have psoriasis, compared with a population frequency of 7%.

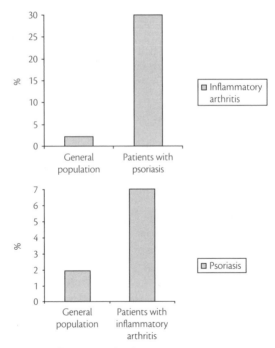

Figure 1.3 Prevalence of psoriasis and arthritis.

Myth

Psoriatic arthritis is an uncommon disease.

 Fact

Psoriatic arthritis may be more common than previously thought and may affect 0.25–0.5% of the population.

Over the past several years, many studies have been carried out to determine the prevalence of psoriatic arthritis. However, these studies used different case definitions and different methods of ascertainment of cases, and the results have been quite varied, with estimates of between 0.001 and 1.5% (Table 1.2). Likewise, the prevalence of psoriatic arthritis among patients with psoriasis has varied between 6 and 42%. Again, the variability depends on the case definition and the methods used to ascertain the cases. The best studies looking at this question identified that approximately 30% of patients with psoriasis develop psoriatic arthritis. Since the usual quoted prevalence of psoriasis in the general population is 2–3%, the prevalence of psoriatic arthritis in the general population should be between 0.6 and 1%.

Manifestations of psoriatic arthritis

Patients with psoriatic arthritis suffer from joint pain and stiffness which are worse following periods of immobility such as sitting for prolonged periods of time or following sleep. Many patients are awakened at night because of joint pain. The affected joints may be swollen, and there may be an associated

Table 1.2 Prevalence of psoriatic arthritis

Population studied	Type of study	Prevalence (%)
Faroe Islands	Population based	1.5
Rochester, USA	Population based	0.1
Japan	Referrals to medical centres	0.001
North-west Greece	Population survey	0.57
Queensland, Australia	Aboriginal survey	1.5

discoloration and heat. Joint pain, stiffness, and swelling often improve with exercise. Any joint may be involved. Common sites include the joints of the feet and hands, the knees, ankles, shoulders, and, less commonly, the hips. These joints are usually referred to as **peripheral joints**. A typical clinical feature of psoriatic arthritis is the involvement of the end joints (**distal joints**) of the fingers and toes, and the **asymmetric distribution** where a joint may be affected on one side of the body but not the other. If the joint inflammation remains untreated it may lead to joint damage with the development of deformities. In psoriatic arthritis, joints may become totally fused, unable to move, or they may become extremely loose and flail.

The joints of the back (spine) are involved in about half of the patients with psoriatic arthritis. This type of arthritis is called **spondylitis**. Spondylitis also presents with pain and stiffness, made worse by inactivity and improving with exercise. Patients may complain of night pain which improves if they get out of bed and walk around or jump into the shower. Upon awakening, the back pain and stiffness often improve with moving around, only to recur with periods of immobility. All parts of the back may be involved, including the neck, the upper back, lower back, and the joints of the pelvis—the **sacroiliac joints**. Back involvement may lead to development of deformities and limitation of movement of the back. Some patients end up with a curved back and marked limitation of neck movements. Back disease often develops late in the course of psoriatic arthritis.

Other features of psoriatic arthritis

In addition to the peripheral joint and back disease associated with psoriatic arthritis, patients with this condition present with swelling of a whole digit, or **dactylitis**. This may occur in half of the patients with psoriatic arthritis. The toes are more likely to be involved than the fingers, but any digit may be affected, and several digits may be affected simultaneously in the same patient. The swollen digit is usually quite painful and is limited in mobility. While the acute pain of dactylitis may resolve without specific treatment, the finger or toe may remain chronically swollen and with limited movement. Dactylitis should be treated immediately if one wishes to preserve normal finger or toe movement.

Another typical feature of psoriatic arthritis is **enthesitis**, or inflammation at the insertion of tendons into bone. This occurs in about 40% of the patients. The most common site of enthesitis is the **Achilles tendon**, at the back of the heel. The **plantar fascia**, at the bottom of the heel, is also commonly affected.

In addition to the skin and joint manifestations of psoriatic arthritis, people with this condition may also develop additional clinical features, called

extra-articular features. These include sores in the mouth as well as inflammation in the eye, either **iritis** or **uveitis**. The latter presents with a red eye, painful to light and associated with blurred vision. Patients may suffer from burning upon passing urine, called **urethritis**. Some patients may have associated diarrhoeal illness which on occasion may become an **inflammatory bowel disease**.

Psoriatic arthritis without psoriasis

Although psoriatic arthritis most often occurs in people with psoriasis, once the clinical picture became clear, it has become possible to make the diagnosis before the psoriasis is detected. We now know that some 15% of patients with psoriatic arthritis develop their arthritis before the appearance of psoriasis. The diagnosis can be made on the basis of the clinical features that are typical for psoriatic arthritis (described above). Many of the patients who present with these typical features who do not have psoriasis may have relatives with psoriasis, and the diagnosis is made easier.

Patterns of psoriatic arthritis

It has now become clear that psoriatic arthritis is a very varied condition. Some patients have only mild enthesitis while others may have severe destructive arthritis affecting many joints. Moll and Wright described five different patterns (Table 1.3). These patterns have been recognized in most large series of patients with psoriatic arthritis.

1. Patients may present with primary involvement of the end joints of the fingers and toes, which are called the distal interphalangeal joints. This pattern is the **distal pattern**, and is noted in fewer than 5% of the patients.

2. Another pattern, where four or less joints are affected, is termed the **oligoarticular pattern**. The oligoarticular pattern often manifests in an

Table 1.3 Patterns of psoriatic arthritis

Distal pattern	Involving primarily the distal joints of the fingers and toes
Oligoarticular pattern	Involving 4 or less peripheral joints
Polyarticular pattern	Involving 5 or more peripheral joints
Spondylitis	Involving primarily the joints of the spine
Arthritis mutilans	A destructive form of arthritis

asymmetric distribution (involvement of joints on one but not the other side of the body), and is very common particularly at disease onset.

3. At least half of the patients with psoriatic arthritis have five or more joints affected, known as the **polyarticular pattern**. This pattern is often asymmetrically distributed, although it is clear that with increasing numbers of joints involved the distribution becomes more symmetric.

4. A fourth pattern of psoriatic arthritis is the back or **spondylitis pattern**. Spondylitis alone, without peripheral arthritis, is uncommon, occurring in 2–4% of patients with psoriatic arthritis. However, in 50% of the patients with peripheral arthritis there is an associated spondylitis. Patients with psoriatic spondylitis may not have any complaints of pain (asymptomatic), in which case it is detected only by X-rays. Other patients with spondylitis may develop a very debilitating form of involvement with marked deformity of the spine and limitation of movement.

5. The fifth pattern, **arthritis mutilans**, is discussed in more detail in Chapter 5.

Over the past few decades, it has become clear that while these patterns are helpful in early disease, they are not helpful in established disease since over time there may be a change in the pattern of psoriatic arthritis. Thus patients who initially present with distal joint disease may develop arthritis in joints at the base of the fingers or toes and therefore no longer qualify for only the distal pattern, or they may develop spondylitis. On the other hand, patients with an initial polyarticular presentation may improve and remain with a small number of joints involved, fitting into the oligoarticular presentation.

Diagnosing psoriatic arthritis

The diagnosis of psoriatic arthritis requires careful assessment by a rheumatologist. The physician usually obtains a detailed history followed by a detailed physical examination. A general physical examination is required, together with a meticulous joint examination to identify the joints affected and the degree of inflammation, as well as the presence of back disease, dactylitis, and enthesitis. Following the clinical examination, laboratory tests are performed. Although there are no specific laboratory abnormalities associated with psoriatic arthritis, these tests are often done to rule out other forms of arthritis, and to obtain a baseline level of liver and kidney function tests prior to starting medications.

Radiographs are often obtained both to confirm the diagnosis and to get a baseline for future disease progression, or the effect of drugs. As in the clinical picture, the X-rays may identify the sites involved, the pattern of involvement, and, if there are changes due to damage, they can be identified as those typical for psoriatic arthritis such as **ankylosis** of some joints or total destruction of others. Radiographs of the back are particularly important since many patients do not complain of back pain yet the presence of **sacroiliitis** or **syndesmophytes** may help make the correct diagnosis.

Diagnostic criteria

Until recently there were no widely accepted criteria for either the classification or diagnosis of psoriatic arthritis. However, an international study was completed in 2006 and resulted in the **ClASs**ification of **P**soriatic **AR**thritis (CASPAR) criteria. The CASPAR criteria should facilitate the diagnosis of the condition. Based on these criteria, if a patient has inflammatory joint disease, inflammatory back disease, or enthesitis, and 3 points collected from a few clinical features, they can be classified and diagnosed as psoriatic arthritis. Thus, if a patient has current psoriasis they get 2 points. If they do not have current psoriasis, but have a history of psoriasis or a family history of psoriasis in a first-degree relative, they get 1 point. The presence of dactylitis, nail lesions, negative rheumatoid factors, and a bony reaction on X-rays each provide 1 point. These criteria were tested in early psoriatic arthritis and in a family practice unit, and are highly sensitive and specific. Therefore, the CASPAR criteria may now be used to classify and possibly diagnose patients with psoriatic arthritis. This will facilitate early detection and hopefully earlier treatment and prevention of joint damage in patients with this disease.

2

The relationship between psoriasis and psoriatic arthritis

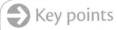

Key points

- Patients with more severe psoriasis may be more likely to develop psoriatic arthritis

- Once psoriatic arthritis is present, there is no direct correlation between the extent and severity of skin and joint manifestations

- Patients with psoriatic arthritis are more likely to have nail lesions than patients with psoriasis without arthritis

Psoriasis in the skin

Psoriasis has diverse manifestations. The most common form is called **psoriasis vulgaris**. Psoriasis vulgaris presents with a plaque often associated with scaling. It can be localized or widespread. It most often affects the extensor surfaces of the knees and elbows (Fig. 2.1, p. 12), as well as the scalp, but may occur anywhere on the body. Psoriasis may also affect flexural areas (**flexural psoriasis**) such as under the arms or breasts, the groins, the genital areas, and the natal cleft. In these areas, it tends to be as thin plaques, often not associated with scales. Some patients develop **guttate psoriasis**, which manifests with multiple small lesions, and others present with **pustular psoriasis**, which look like whiteheads, and often occur on the palms and soles, but at times may be quite widespread. Guttate psoriasis often occurs after an upper respiratory tract infection with *Streptococcus* ('strep. throat').

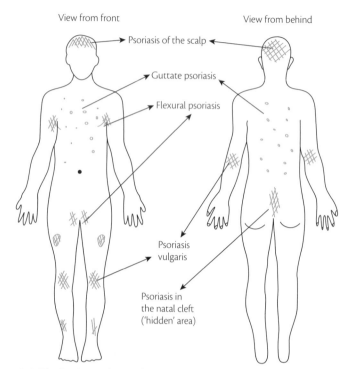

View from front   View from behind

Psoriasis of the scalp

Guttate psoriasis

Flexural psoriasis

Psoriasis
vulgaris

Psoriasis in
the natal cleft
('hidden' area)

Figure 2.1 Distribution and type of psoriasis.

Psoriatic nail lesions

Nail lesions are common in psoriasis, manifesting as small indentations in the nail plate (**nail pitting**); separation of the nail from its bed (**onycholysis**); light brown translucent patches under the nail plate (oil drops); or thickening of the nail plate with hyperkeratosis of the nail bed (**subungual hyperkeratosis**) (Fig. 2.2, p. 13). The extent may vary from a few nails to all finger and toe nails. Sometimes it is difficult to distinguish psoriatic nail changes from fungal infection, particularly in the toes.

Skin and joint manifestations at presentation

The majority of patients with psoriatic arthritis present with the skin disease prior to or at the same time as the development of the arthritis. However, the relationship between the skin and joint manifestations remains unclear. Most studies reporting on series of patients with psoriatic arthritis describe

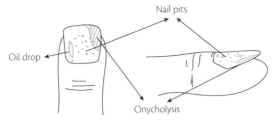

Figure 2.2 Typical changes seen on the nails in psoriasis.

between 15 and 20% of the patients whose arthritis was diagnosed before the detection of the skin psoriasis. In some of the patients who present with psoriatic arthritis before the onset of skin disease, the psoriasis may be missed. People often do not recognize the scaly lesions as psoriasis, and do not show the rash to their doctor. The skin lesions may be hidden in places such as the umbilical area or the anal (natal) cleft, sites that are not easily detected by the patients. Sometimes the psoriasis is only present at the hairline at the back, or behind the ears, areas which are also not seen by the patient. When patients see a physician, they do not necessarily complain of their skin lesions as they do not know about the relationship between the skin lesions and arthritis. If the physician does not get the patient totally undressed to check their skin carefully for any presence of psoriatic skin lesions, particularly in these 'hidden' areas, they might miss the diagnosis of psoriasis, and may not make the correct diagnosis of psoriatic arthritis.

Do only patients with severe psoriasis get arthritis?

Early reports suggested that psoriatic arthritis was associated with severe psoriasis. This was based on a few series of patients hospitalized for psoriasis, where the prevalence of psoriatic arthritis was 30%. It was therefore thought that since patients are admitted to hospital because of psoriasis when the psoriasis is severe, then the arthritis was associated with severe psoriasis. Since earlier reports suggested the prevalence of psoriatic arthritis among patients with psoriasis to be only 7%, it appeared that patients whose psoriasis was severe enough for them to be hospitalized were more likely to develop psoriatic arthritis. However, it became clear that even in outpatient dermatology clinics the prevalence of arthritis could be as high as 42%. Moreover, the fact that up to 20% of patients with clinical symptoms highly suggestive of psoriatic arthritis have no psoriasis at onset suggests that there is no direct relationship between the extent or severity of psoriasis and the development of the arthritis.

National Psoriasis Foundation survey

A survey by the National Psoriasis Foundation in the USA found that the prevalence of arthritis among patients with psoriasis was 11%. In the survey, patients were asked about the extent of their psoriasis. This was done on the basis of the number of the patient's palms required to describe the extent of psoriasis. It is usually considered that the palm represents 1% of the body surface area. Thus less than one palm is very mild and more than ten palms is considered very severe. On the basis of this estimation of the severity of the psoriasis, patients with very little psoriasis had a frequency of psoriatic arthritis of only 6% while those who had more than ten palms had a 56% frequency of psoriatic arthritis. This study thus supports the notion that people with more extensive psoriasis are more likely to suffer from psoriatic arthritis. However, a similar survey performed in Europe provided a prevalence of arthritis among patients with psoriasis of 30%, and the association with more extensive disease was not noted.

 Myth

Psoriatic arthritis occurs in patients with severe psoriasis.

 Fact

While the severity of psoriasis may be related to the development of psoriatic arthritis in the first place, once there, there is no direct relationship between the severity of skin and joint manifestations.

Severity of skin and joint manifestations over the course of the disease

Once psoriatic arthritis has been diagnosed, there appears to be little correlation between the severity of the arthritis and the severity and/or distribution of skin disease. In a large prospective study from Toronto, Canada, only a third of the patients recognized a relationship between skin and joint flares. A study that included 221 patients with psoriatic arthritis who participated in a randomized controlled trial showed that there was no correlation between the extent of joint disease measured by the **actively inflamed joint count** (number of swollen and/or tender joints) and the severity of skin disease measured by the psoriasis area and severity index **(PASI)**. Another study of 71 patients suggested that while overall there was no relationship between skin and joint disease, in those patients who presented with skin and joint manifestations simultaneously, there was a correlation. In the Toronto clinic, there was also no correlation between actively inflamed joint count and PASI scores over time.

Thus, while the predisposition to the development of arthritis may be related to the extent of psoriasis, the severity of joint disease does not appear to be related to the severity of skin disease, and vice versa. Nonetheless, when treating patients with psoriatic arthritis, physicians pay attention to both skin and joint manifestations and attempt to control both aspects of the disease by using medications that work for both.

Psoriatic nail lesions and psoriatic arthritis

The presence of nail lesions does correlate with the presence of psoriatic arthritis among patients with psoriasis. However, the type of nail lesion does not correlate with the presence of arthritis, as all nail lesions described above have been noted both among patients with uncomplicated psoriasis and in those with psoriatic arthritis. In a study that compared 158 patients with psoriatic arthritis with 101 patients with psoriasis without arthritis, the only clinical feature that differentiated the two groups was the presence of nail lesions. Nail lesions occurred in 46% of patients with uncomplicated psoriasis and in 87% of patients with psoriatic arthritis. Nail lesions are particularly common in patients with involvement of the end joints (distal joints) of the fingers and toes. Indeed, some patients with psoriatic arthritis have had only nail lesions, without any other evidence of skin psoriasis. The ClASsification of Psoriatic ARthritis (CASPAR) criteria that were developed through an international effort allow the diagnosis of psoriatic arthritis to be made in the absence of psoriatic skin lesions if nail lesions are present.

Relationship between skin and joint manifestations
Skin and joint severity relationship

The relationship between psoriasis and its associated arthritis may be described as four quadrants, depending on the extent of skin and joint disease (Fig. 2.3, p. 16). In one quadrant there will be patients with very mild psoriasis and mild arthritis. These patients may or may not be referred to a specialist, be it a dermatologist or a rheumatologist. In another quadrant there will be patients with very severe psoriasis but mild arthritis. These patients are more likely to see a dermatologist, and may or may not be referred to a rheumatologist. In the third quadrant there will be patients with mild psoriasis and severe arthritis.

These patients are more likely to be referred to a rheumatologist, but may not be seen by a dermatologist. In the final quadrant there will be patients with severe psoriasis and severe arthritis. These patients are most likely to be seen by both a rheumatologist and a dermatologist. At the top of this relationship there will be patients with psoriasis without any arthritis at all, and at the bottom, there will be patients with arthritis but without psoriasis. Of all patients with psoriasis, we know that about 30% will have psoriatic arthritis. Thus, of all patients with psoriasis there will be about 70% who will not develop arthritis. Of all patients with psoriatic arthritis we know that about 15–20% will develop the arthritis before developing the psoriasis. The exact relationship within the four quadrants is not yet known since we do not have a clear picture of the totality of psoriatic arthritis.

 Myth

Psoriatic arthritis occurs only in patients with psoriasis.

Fact

Psoriatic arthritis may develop in patients without psoriasis. The psoriasis may develop later. Close relatives of these patients may have psoriasis.

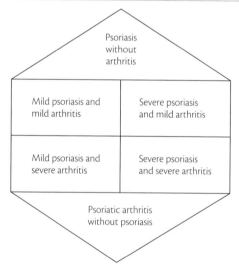

Figure 2.3 Relationship between psoriasis and psoriatic arthritis.

Summary

It is recommended that all patients with mild psoriasis be seen by a dermatologist who should be able to determine whether there is a possibility of psoriatic arthritis. The dermatologist would then refer such patients to a rheumatologist. Likewise, if a patient is referred to a rheumatologist with what turns out to be psoriatic arthritis, they should be referred to a dermatologist to confirm the diagnosis and help with the management of the psoriasis. Only when dermatologists and rheumatologists work together as a team will we be able to determine the exact relationship between psoriatic skin and joint disease.

3

Psoriatic arthritis and other spondyloarthritides

> ## ➔ Key points

> ◆ Spondyloarthritides are a group of inflammatory arthritis conditions that share the involvement of the spine as well as other specific features

> ◆ Spondyloarthritides are different from rheumatoid arthritis

> ◆ Psoriatic arthritis is a form of spondyloarthritides distinguishable by its clinical features

As described in the two preceding chapters, psoriatic arthritis is not just the occurrence of 'arthritis' with psoriasis. In fact, psoriatic arthritis is a specific inflammatory arthritis that occurs in people with psoriasis. Psoriatic arthritis has a number of specific features that help in making a diagnosis. In fact, psoriatic arthritis can even be diagnosed in the absence of psoriasis.

Inflammatory and degenerative arthritis

Arthritis in general can be separated into two major classes—inflammatory and degenerative (Fig. 3.1, p. 20). Degenerative arthritis, also called osteoarthritis, is the most common type of arthritis and is believed to be due to 'wear and tear' of the joints. Osteoarthritis affects weight-bearing joints such as the hips, knees, and joints in the neck and low back, and this type of arthritis is associated with increasing age and previous injuries. The other class of arthritis is called inflammatory arthritis. Here, joint inflammation due to an inciting agent affects primarily the lining of the joint rather than causing wear and tear, and leads to joint damage. Inflammatory arthritis may be grouped into two major groups—that due to a specific cause ('known' cause) and that due to an unknown cause, or 'idiopathic'. Joint inflammation may be triggered by known agents. When triggered by infectious agents such as viruses or bacteria, it is termed infectious arthritis. Other causes include arthritis triggered by crystals, such as uric acid (gout) and calcium pyrophosphate (pseudogout).

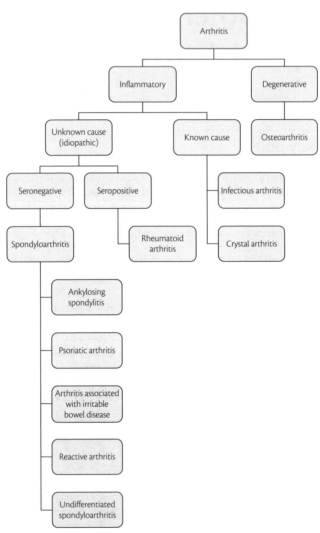

Figure 3.1 A simple classification of arthritides.

When the cause of inflammatory arthritis is not clearly evident, it is termed idiopathic. It is believed that genetic and environmental factors interact to trigger joint inflammation. Idiopathic inflammatory arthritis can be simplistically classified into seropositive and seronegative. This classification is based on the presence of a protein in the blood called rheumatoid factor. Most patients with idiopathic inflammatory arthritis who test positive for the rheumatoid factor have rheumatoid arthritis. Those who do not test positive for rheumatoid factor have seronegative spondyloarthritis. Psoriatic arthritis belongs to the seronegative spondyloarthritis class of idiopathic inflammatory arthritis.

Seronegative spondyloarthritides

Seronegative spondyloarthritides are a group of closely related inflammatory diseases that were first distinguished from rheumatoid arthritis after the rheumatoid factor was discovered in 1948, although they had important clinical differences. Further distinction of this class of arthritis occurred after the discovery of a gene called HLA-B27. Just as most patients with rheumatoid arthritis test positive for rheumatoid factor, most patients with seronegative spondyloarthritis test positive for the HLA-B27 gene. Thus, these tests in conjunction with careful clinical evaluation help the physician to distinguish between rheumatoid arthritis and seronegative spondyloarthritides. However, these tests by themselves are not diagnostic.

A number of arthritic conditions belong to the class of seronegative spondyloarthritides. The members include ankylosing spondylitis, psoriatic arthritis, reactive arthritis, arthritis associated with inflammatory bowel disease, juvenile spondyloarthritis, and undifferentiated spondyloarthritis. These arthritic conditions are grouped together as they have a set of common features that distinguishes them from rheumatoid arthritis.

Inflammation in the joints of the back and neck (axial arthritis) is the characteristic feature of seronegative spondyloarthritides. The axial joints that are involved include the sacroiliac joints (the joints between the sacrum and iliac bones) and the joints between the various vertebrae in the lumbar, thoracic, and cervical spine. Inflammatory back pain is the characteristic symptom of axial inflammatory arthritis (spondyloarthritis). This manifests clinically as pain in the low back, or neck and buttock pain associated with prolonged stiffness that is often felt after periods of prolonged rest, especially during the second half of the night and early morning. Pain and stiffness tend to improve with activity. In contrast, mechanical back pain improves with rest and is worse after activity. Gradually, there is fusion of the vertebrae to one another, leading to restricted mobility. Rheumatoid arthritis does not involve the sacroiliac joints or lower spinal vertebral joints.

Inflammation of the joints of the extremities (peripheral arthritis) is, in general, less common in seronegative spondyloarthritis compared with seropositive disease. Characteristically, peripheral arthritis occurs in the lower limb joints, is asymmetric, and involves four joints or less. This is in contrast to rheumatoid arthritis, which usually involves five or more joints, is symmetric, and predominantly involves joints of the upper limbs. Deformities seen classically in rheumatoid arthritis are usually not seen among the spondyloarthritis group of conditions. Radiographic evidence of damage is less pronounced than in rheumatoid arthritis, although there can be considerable peripheral joint damage in psoriatic arthritis, and damage to hip joints is more frequently seen in ankylosing spondylitis.

Another distinguishing feature of seronegative spondyloarthritides is inflammation at sites of insertion of tendons and ligaments (entheses), known as enthesitis. Indeed, some experts believe that the primary pathology in seronegative spondyloarthritis is enthesitis. Another important feature that differentiates seronegative spondyloarthritis from rheumatoid arthritis is dactylitis, commonly known as 'sausage digits'. Dactylitis is the swelling of the entire finger or toe due to inflammation. Dactylitis results from the swelling of the tendons, soft tissue, bone, and joints.

Other important features of these diseases are the manifestations at sites other than the joints, so called extra-articular manifestations. These manifestations involve the skin, mucous membranes, and eyes. Patients with psoriatic arthritis have psoriasis and those with arthritis associated with inflammatory bowel diseases have inflammatory bowel disease. Inflammation in the eye is particularly characteristic, manifesting as inflammation of the conjunctiva (conjunctivitis) or inflammation of the uvea (uveitis).

How is psoriatic arthritis different from other spondyloarthritides?

The defining feature of psoriatic arthritis is the presence of psoriasis affecting the skin and nails. The arthritis usually manifests after the psoriasis begins, but sometimes can precede the psoriasis. Psoriatic arthritis has a number of features that distinguish it from other seronegative spondyloarthritides. The peripheral joints are usually involved and it is often polyarticular, especially in long-standing disease. Peripheral arthritis frequently involves upper limb joints, and can sometimes mimic rheumatoid arthritis especially when it is symmetric. Joint damage is frequent and can lead to deformities. Enthesitis and dactylitis are frequent. The axial involvement in psoriatic arthritis differs from that in ankylosing spondylitis in being less symptomatic (less painful and stiff) and less symmetric on X-rays (there are differences between the two sides of the body). Thus, although psoriatic arthritis has a number of features in common with the other seronegative spondyloarthritides, it can be distinguished by a number of characteristic features. These features will be discussed in subsequent chapters.

Thus, to summarize, psoriatic arthritis is an inflammatory arthritis associated with psoriasis that belongs to a class of arthritis called seronegative spondyloarthritides which can be distinguished from rheumatoid arthritis. There are a number of features that distinguishes psoriatic arthritis from other seronegative spondyloarthritides, principally psoriasis and the pattern of peripheral arthritis.

4

What causes psoriatic arthritis

→ Key points

◆ Psoriatic arthritis is a complex genetic disease

◆ Environmental factors make a significant contribution to its development

◆ Psoriatic arthritis is an immune-mediated inflammatory disease

Psoriatic arthritis is a complex disease. There are genetic, environmental, and immunological factors involved in the onset and progression of psoriatic arthritis (Fig. 4.1, p. 26). In this chapter, we have made an attempt to describe our understanding of these factors.

Psoriatic arthritis is an immune-mediated inflammatory disease that primarily affects the skin, the joints, and related structures. It is believed that environmental factors initiate immunological processes in a genetically susceptible individual. We shall first describe the current knowledge of genetic factors and possible environmental triggers, and then the mechanisms that operate in joint inflammation and damage.

Genetic factors

It is believed that susceptibility to most human diseases is influenced by genetic (hereditary) and environmental factors. Inherited diseases such as cystic fibrosis or sickle cell disease have a large genetic component with a minor contribution from environmental factors. These two diseases are mediated through a mutation of a single gene (**simple genetic diseases**). On the other hand,

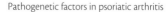

Pathogenetic factors in psoriatic arthritis

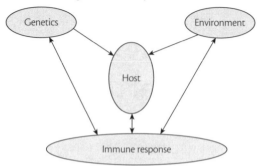

Figure 4.1 Inter-relationship between genetic, environmental, and immunological factors in psoriatic arthritis.

infectious diseases such as acquired immunodeficiency syndrome (AIDS) and tuberculosis have a large environmental component, the genetic component being relatively minor. Most other diseases, especially **autoimmune diseases**, have a significant contribution from both genetic and environmental factors. In these conditions, a number of different genes contribute to susceptibility, and these are often called **complex genetic disease**.

How does one study whether genetic factors are indeed important in a disease?

Family studies

The first step in identifying the role of genetic factors in disease is to study the presence of the disease in families and to determine whether there is increased prevalence among family members as compared with the general population. Studying identical and non-identical twins is another strategy to determine the genetic contribution to a disease. Unfortunately, there have been few studies to determine whether there is an increased prevalence of psoriatic arthritis in families. Studies done in the UK have shown that close relatives of patients with psoriatic arthritis have 55 times the risk of developing psoriatic arthritis compared with the general population. Our own studies, conducted in Canada, have shown similar results, although the magnitude of the risk is smaller, being close to 30. Until recently, there have been no twin studies conducted in psoriatic arthritis. A recent study from Denmark demonstrated the occurrence of psoriasis among identical twins, but only one of ten identical twins sets were concordant of psoriatic arthritis. This means that environmental factors may play a significant role in the development of psoriatic arthritis. However, it is clear that there is indeed a greatly increased risk in close relatives of patients with psoriatic arthritis mostly due to genetic factors. Interestingly, we have also shown that the risk of transmitting psoriatic arthritis is higher if the affected parent is the father. This indicates that there are modifying factors on the heritable gene (**epigenetic factors**) which are also involved in making one susceptible to psoriatic arthritis.

Genetic linkage studies

Once genetic factors are suspected to play an important role in a disease, the next step is to conduct **genetic linkage studies**. Linkage studies are done by collecting information on families with affected members. DNA is tested using a set of markers that span the genome at equal intervals. Linkage studies provide information on the possible regions of interest on the human genome where genes causing the disease might be located. When a region is located, by comparing affected and non-affected individuals, further studies are done. These studies include fine-mapping of the areas of interest to try and identify the actual gene involved. Only one such study has been conducted in psoriatic arthritis, and a region on chromosome 16 was identified as a region of interest.

Genetic association studies

Another way to detect genes associated with a disease is by conducting **genetic association studies**. Association studies are done by comparing a large number of carefully studied patients with an equal number of normal subjects who are matched by age, sex, and ethnicity. A number of genes have been shown to be associated with psoriatic arthritis and some of them have been confirmed by a different group of researchers. Those genes that have been shown consistently to be associated with psoriatic arthritis will be reviewed here.

Human leukocyte antigen (HLA) genes

HLA genes on chromosome 6 were found to be associated with psoriatic arthritis more than 30 years ago. HLA genes are classified into class I and class II. HLA A, B, and C belong to class I, whereas HLA DP, DQ, and DR belong to class II. HLA genes code for antigens present on the surface of cells in the body, especially cells of the immune system. Antigens produced by HLA class I genes are present on almost all cells of the body, whereas those produced by HLA class II genes are present mainly on immune cells.

Class I antigens (HLA-B13, HLA-B57, HLA-B39, HLA-Cw6, and HLA-Cw7) were shown to be associated with psoriasis and psoriatic arthritis by many researchers worldwide. The strongest association is with HLA-Cw6. HLA class I antigens have also been associated with various types of psoriatic arthritis. HLA-B27 is associated with back disease, and HLA-B38 and HLA-B39 with peripheral arthritis. Class II antigens have not been found to be associated with psoriatic arthritis, although in individuals with psoriatic arthritis they may influence how the disease expresses itself. For example, a group of class II antigens that is well known to cause severe disease in rheumatoid arthritis may cause severe disease in psoriatic arthritis. Recently, patients with psoriatic arthritis carrying both HLA-Cw6 and HLA-DR7 genes were found to have a less severe course of arthritis. However, although these associations were discovered many years ago and these genes are markers of disease, how they cause disease or affect disease expression has not been discovered yet. It is possible that genes lying close to these genes on chromosome 6 are the 'real' culprits. Moreover, although there is a clear association between psoriatic arthritis and the HLA genes, these are not present in all patients who have the disease. Therefore, there must be other genes which are important in the development of psoriatic arthritis.

Killer cell immunoglobulin receptor (KIR) genes

To explain the possible mechanisms of how HLA class I genes increase susceptibility to psoriatic arthritis, researchers have investigated a set of genes on chromosome 19 called killer cell immunoglobulin receptor (KIR) genes. The protein produced by this gene is a receptor that is present on important cells of the immune system—the natural killer or NK cells and NK-T cells. NK cells are important cells in the initial contact with insulting agents. NK cells have a role in the inflammatory response in psoriasis and psoriatic arthritis. In order for the NK receptor to be activated, it has to interact with HLA-C antigen on the surface of the cell. Therefore, HLA-C is considered to be the **ligand** for KIR. Interaction between HLA-C antigen on cells and the KIRs can therefore modulate the immune response. KIRs are of two types, activating and inhibitory. Inheritance of certain activating KIRs, particularly KIR2DS1 and KIR2DS2, has been found to be associated with psoriasis and psoriatic arthritis, and lack of inhibitory KIRs or their corresponding HLA-C ligand has been shown to be associated with the development of psoriatic arthritis. Further research into the KIR genes and their interaction with HLA in psoriatic arthritis will shed light on these intriguing systems of genes.

Tumour necrosis factor-α (TNF-α) and class I major histocompatibility complex chain-related gene A (MICA)

How HLA genes increase the risk for psoriatic arthritis is unknown. Interaction with KIR genes is a plausible explanation. Another explanation is that it is not HLA genes *per se* that are responsible, but other genes lying close to the HLA genes on chromosome 6. Two such genes that have been shown to lie close to HLA genes and are associated with psoriatic arthritis are TNF-α and MICA genes.

The TNF-α gene was found to be associated with psoriatic arthritis by a number of researchers. This gene lies within the area where the HLA genes are located on chromosome 6. The TNF-α gene controls the production of TNF-α protein which is an important molecule that causes inflammation in psoriatic arthritis. Blocking this protein using drugs called anti-TNF-α agents causes marked reduction in inflammation in both the joints and the skin, and also prevents further damage to the joints. There is a variant of the gene which is more common among patients with psoriatic arthritis than healthy controls. Another gene, the MICA gene, located within the HLA region, has also been shown to be associated with psoriatic arthritis by a number of researchers. The MICA gene produces a protein called MICA that associates with HLA class I antigens on the surface of most cells of the body. MICA is also important in NK cell activation since it is the ligand for a receptor on NK cells called NKG2D. Thus, MICA is also important in the immune response and may play a role in the development of psoriatic arthritis. Clearly, this region of our chromosome needs to be investigated further before definite conclusions can be drawn.

Genes outside chromosome 6, other than KIR genes on chromosome 19, have also been investigated for association with psoriatic arthritis. However, after initial identification, only a handful of genes have been confirmed by another independent group of researchers. The interleukin-1 (IL-1) gene on chromosome 2q was found to be associated with psoriatic arthritis. Recently, the interleukin-23 (IL-23) receptor gene was also found to be associated with psoriatic arthritis. This particular gene is also important in psoriasis. Both these genes code for proteins involved in the immune response.

Environmental factors

Genetic factors cannot fully explain an individual's susceptibility to psoriatic arthritis. Environmental factors are probably involved, as in other complex diseases. It is likely that environmental factors trigger the illness in a genetically susceptible individual. However, no single agent has been clearly identified. Physical trauma is one such environmental factor. There are reports of onset of psoriatic arthritis after significant injury to joints. Viral infections may also trigger psoriatic arthritis. It is well known that patients with human immuno-deficiency virus (HIV) infection that causes AIDS have severe psoriasis and psoriatic arthritis. Recently, rubella vaccination, injury sufficient to require a medical consultation, a fractured bone, and moving house were found to be associated with onset of psoriatic arthritis. Large-scale systematic studies to identify such environmental factors have not yet been done.

Immunological factors

Psoriatic arthritis is an immune-mediated inflammatory disease. Environmental factors probably initiate an inappropriate immune response in a genetically susceptible individual. As described above, most genes that are associated with psoriatic arthritis code for proteins involved in the immune response.

Immune-mediated processes that initiate and perpetuate the immune response have two arms—the antibody-mediated response arm and the cell-mediated response arm. The antibody arm does not seem to play an important role in psoriatic arthritis because **autoantibodies** have not been identified in the blood of patients with psoriatic arthritis. The major player in psoriatic arthritis is the cell-mediated immune response. **T cells**, and particularly a group called CD8+ T cells, are important. These cells have been found to be increased in the affected skin as well as in the joint fluid of arthritic joints in patients with psoriatic arthritis. Drugs that block T cells, such as cyclosporin, efaluzimab, and alefacept, are known to improve joint inflammation.

What drives the immune response in the psoriatic joint?

Activated T cells produce pro-inflammatory factors called **cytokines** that drive the inappropriate immune response. The T cells that are important belong to the Th-1 pathway of T helper cells. These cells are important in the cell-mediated immune response. Recently, a new pathway of T helper cell-mediated inflammation called the Th-17 pathway has been discovered. Important cytokines that drive the immune response in psoriatic arthritis joints include TNF-α and IL-1. The cytokines that mediate the Th-17 pathway include IL-17 and IL-23. The Th-17 pathway is important in mediating a number of inflammatory diseases such as psoriasis, rheumatoid arthritis, and inflammatory bowel disease. It is likely that the same pathway is important in psoriatic arthritis. An environmental trigger such as a viral or bacterial infection or trauma (micro-trauma or overt trauma) initiates the cell-mediated Th-1/Th-17 pathway in the psoriatic joint. The immune response in the joint activates T cells, and these cells mediate the secretion of these pro-inflammatory cytokines. Cytokines such as TNF-α and IL-23 are important in mediating the disease because both skin and joint inflammation is ameliorated by drug therapy that blocks TNF-α and IL-23.

Analysis of T cells in the fluid in psoriatic joints has shown a predominance of mature and activated T cells. Cytokines such as TNF-α and IL-1 are increased in the joint fluid and the joint lining. Activated T cells also produce inflammatory molecules called receptor activator for NF-κB ligand (RANKL) that activate bone-destroying cells called **osteoclasts**. These osteoclasts then eat away bone close to the joint, causing joint destruction. An important feature of psoriatic arthritis that distinguishes it from rheumatoid arthritis is new bone formation at sites of inflammation. Thus psoriatic arthritis destroys bone and also leads to abnormal new bone formation at these sites. It is possible that the wnt signalling pathway whose mediator is dikkopf-1 is an important mediator of new bone formation in psoriatic arthritis.

Thus, to summarize, we believe that an environmental trigger initiates an immune response in the skin and joints of genetically predisposed patients with psoriatic arthritis. The immune response is initiated involving the Th-1/Th-17 pathway of T helper cells. These immune cells initiate an inflammatory reaction and secrete cytokines that activate other inflammatory cells that cause joint damage. These cells also activate osteoclasts that damage neighbouring bone. They also lead to new bone formation, which is characteristic of psoriatic arthritis.

5

Clinical features of psoriatic arthritis

> **Key points**

- There are several important features to psoriatic arthritis

  - Peripheral arthritis

  - Spine involvement

  - Dactylitis

  - Enthesitis

  - Skin and nail involvement

- There are specific extra-articular features

- There are important co-morbidities

- Psoriatic arthritis is associated with increased mortality

Psoriatic arthritis is defined as inflammatory arthritis associated with psoriasis, usually negative for rheumatoid factor. This statement essentially summarizes the clinical features of the psoriatic arthritis. The primary clinical feature is inflammatory arthritis; inflammatory arthritis presents with pain, swelling, stiffness, redness, and often reduction in mobility. In psoriatic arthritis, in addition to the inflammatory arthritis, there are a number of other associated features that makes this arthritic condition unique. These manifestations will be reviewed in this chapter.

Peripheral arthritis

The arthritis of psoriatic arthritis usually begins gradually and involves one or more joints. It often affects the joints in the lower limbs, but any joint of the body may be affected (Fig 5.1). Within a short period, a number of joints are involved. The symptoms of inflammatory arthritis include pain, swelling, and stiffness (Fig 5.2, page 35). Joints that are typically affected in patients with psoriatic arthritis include the end joints of the fingers and toes (distal joints). Commonly the fingernails of these affected joints demonstrate the nail changes that are typical for psoriasis. The distribution of the joint involvement in psoriatic arthritis is often asymmetric—the same joints are not involved in both sides of the body. However, as the number of joints affected increases, there is a tendency towards symmetry.

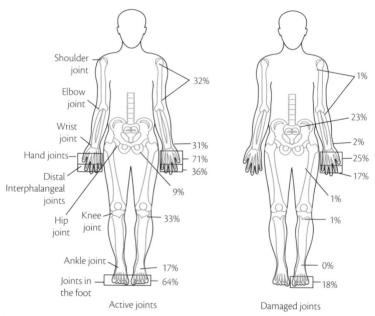

Figure 5.1 Distribution of joint involvement in psoriatic arthritis at presentation (data from the University of Toronto Psoriatic Arthritis Clinic).

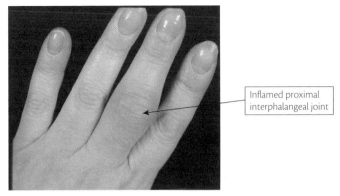

Inflamed proximal interphalangeal joint

Figure 5.2 Actively inflamed joint.

Consequences of peripheral arthritis

The pain and stiffness lead to limitation in movement of the joint. This can lead to limitation in activities of daily living that the person suffering from psoriatic arthritis undertakes. Interestingly, it has been shown that patients with psoriatic arthritis have less pain than those with rheumatoid arthritis. Therefore, they may be oblivious to the degree of inflammation in their joint. Persistent untreated inflammation leads to joint damage. Joint damage manifests clinically as a decrease in range of motion of the joint and development of deformities (Fig. 5.3).

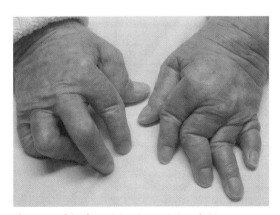

Figure 5.3 Deformities of the finger joints in psoriatic arthritis.

Myth

Psoriatic arthritis is a mild disease.

Fact

Psoriatic arthritis can lead to destructive arthritis of peripheral joints, and fusion and deformity of spinal joints. Patients are also at an increased risk of death compared with the general population, the number of years lost due to the disease being about 3 years on average.

Spondylitis

In addition to the arthritis in the peripheral joints (the joints of the hands and feet), psoriatic arthritis can also affect the joints in the back (so-called axial skeleton). Inflammatory arthritis of the back or neck, technically called spondyloarthritis, causes back or neck pain. The back or neck pain is typically associated with stiffness and is worse after periods of rest, especially after sleep. The pain and stiffness can be so severe as to wake one up in the latter half of the night. The pain and stiffness improve gradually with activity and after a hot shower. Persistent inflammation in the joints of the back may lead to marked restriction in the mobility of the spine (neck and back), making it difficult to turn one's neck or to bend forward or sideways. Ultimately, the process can lead to a completely fused and immobile spine, sometimes called 'bamboo spine' (Fig. 5.4, p. 37).

Dactylitis

Another major manifestation that is characteristic of psoriatic arthritis is dactylitis. Dactylitis, commonly known as 'sausage digit', is defined as inflammatory swelling of an entire finger or toe. This is due to inflammation of the joints, tendons, bones, and soft tissues in the finger or toe. Persistent dactylitis leads to destruction of the joints in that digit. Consequently the finger or toe becomes non-functional. Dactylitis is therefore a marker of severity of psoriatic arthritis (Fig. 5.5).

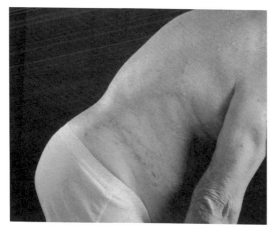

Figure 5.4 Restricted spinal mobility due to involvement of the spine in psoriatic arthritis (psoriatic spondylitis).

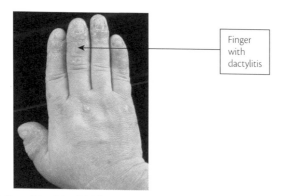

Finger
with
dactylitis

Figure 5.5 Dactylitis of the third finger in psoriatic arthritis.

Enthesitis

Enthesitis is another important manifestation of psoriatic arthritis. In fact, some researchers believe that enthesitis is the primary manifestation of psoriatic arthritis. Enthesitis is defined as inflammation at the site where ligaments or tendons attach to bone. Patients present with pain and swelling in these sites.

The most common sites to be affected by enthesitis are the plantar fascia on the soles of the feet (called plantar fasciitis) and Achilles tendon insertion at the back of the heel (Fig. 5.6). Enthesitis can also affect other sites including tendon insertion sites around the knees and knee caps, shoulders, elbows, sides of the hips, ischial tuberosity (the bone deep in the buttocks that one sits on), and the chest wall.

Tendonitis

Other manifestations include tenosynovitis defined as inflammation of the tendon sheath. Tendons in the hands are usually involved and moving the finger can be painful. Painful thickening of the tendon sheath can be felt on examination. Tenosynovitis can lead to a stiff finger or a 'trigger' finger. The finger gets 'stuck' in a particular position on bending and can be straightened only after applying some amount of force. A snapping sound is heard when the finger is forcibly straightened. Tendon sheaths around the wrists and ankles may also be involved, causing pain on movement of the wrists or ankles.

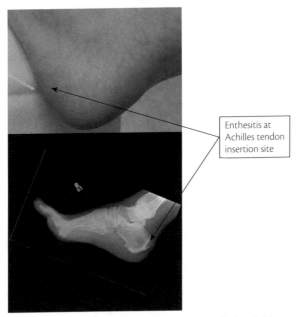

Enthesitis at Achilles tendon insertion site

Figure 5.6 Enthesitis at the Achilles tendon insertion in psoriatic arthritis.

Myth

Psoriatic arthritis affects joints only.

Fact

Psoriatic arthritis affects joints in the extremities and the spine, and also closely related structures such as the entheses and tendon sheaths. Other affected areas include skin, nails, eyes, and intestines. In fact some researchers refer to it as psoriatic disease.

Patterns of psoriatic arthritis

Various patterns of arthritis have been described in psoriatic arthritis. The five patterns originally described by Moll and Wright, who are considered to be pioneers in describing this condition, include:

- Asymmetric oligoarthritis

- Symmetric polyarthritis similar to rheumatoid arthritis

- Spondyloarthritis

- Distal interphalangeal joint arthritis

- Arthritis mutilans

The category of asymmetric oligoarthritis includes those patients with four joints or less affected by arthritis. The joints involved are usually of the lower limbs and there is lack of symmetry. In the category of symmetric polyarthritis, five or more joints are involved in a symmetric fashion. Therefore, it is sometimes difficult to distinguish it from rheumatoid arthritis. The spondyloarthritis category includes patients with predominant involvement of the spine, similar to the involvement in patients with ankylosing spondylitis. As the name suggests, the category of distal interphalangeal joint arthritis includes those patients with predominant involvement of the distal interphalangeal joints, the joint that is at the end of the fingers and toes, closest to the nails (Fig. 5.7, p. 40). Arthritis mutilans describes a category with severe arthritis leading to shortening and destruction of fingers and toes (Fig. 5.8).

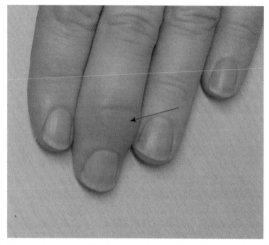

Figure 5.7 Inflammation at the distal interphalangeal joint in psoriatic arthritis.

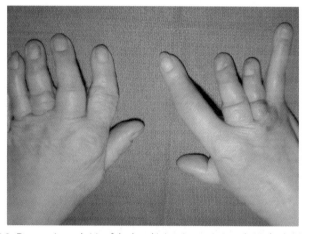

Figure 5.8 Destructive arthritis of the hand joints in psoriatic arthritis (arthritis mutilans).

Myth

Patients presenting with one of the five patterns of psoriatic arthritis tend to maintain that pattern.

Fact

Psoriatic arthritis may initially have a particular pattern, but soon evolves into another; therefore, psoriatic arthritis may be classified into three patterns—peripheral, axial, or both peripheral and axial.

Although initially thought to be distinct patterns, it was soon realized that as the duration of disease increases, the number of joints involved increases and the involvement becomes more symmetric. Distal joint involvement is also common and is seen in all categories. Arthritis mutilans is a manifestation of severity of the arthritis process and not an exclusive category. Therefore, experts nowadays tend to classify the disease as peripheral arthritis alone, peripheral arthritis with spondyloarthritis, and spondyloarthritis alone.

Skin involvement

Most patients with psoriatic arthritis have cutaneous psoriasis. Psoriatic skin disease can be of many types. The most common type is called psoriasis vulgaris, in which the psoriatic skin lesions develop and persist on the scalp, trunk, and extremities, especially on the outer aspects. Inverse or flexurab psoriasis describes the predominant presence of psoriasis on the body folds, especially groin, armpits, and below the breast. Psoriasis can also manifest as a large number of small rounded spots especially on the trunk. This pattern is called guttate psoriasis and it often occurs as a manifestation of worsening psoriasis in patients with other forms of psoriasis, especially after streptococcal infection of the throat ('strep. throat'). Psoriasis may sometimes involve only the hands and/or feet. Severe forms of psoriasis include psoriatic erythroderma when almost the entire body is covered with psoriasis, or when most areas of the body are covered with a small pus-laden skin rash—pustular psoriasis. Both these forms of psoriasis can be life-threatening and require urgent medical attention.

Most patients with psoriatic arthritis have psoriasis vulgaris. In about 70% of people with psoriatic arthritis, psoriasis develops first and the arthritis manifests itself after a variable duration, usually within 10 years. However, this is not always the case. In about 15% of patients, both arthritis and psoriasis develop simultaneously, and in the remainder the arthritis develops first, and cutaneous psoriasis manifests itself a few years later. Some experts believe that patients with more extensive psoriasis tend to develop psoriatic arthritis. This is based on studies on patients hospitalized for severe psoriasis in whom a prevalence of psoriatic arthritis was recorded. A recent survey done through telephone interview reported a higher prevalence of psoriatic arthritis in patients reporting greater extent of psoriasis. However, most patients attending rheumatology clinics for their arthritis have only mild to moderate psoriasis.

Nail involvement

Psoriasis can involve fingernails and toenails. The nails affected by psoriasis have pits, are thickened, and have a yellowish discoloration. The nail may be lifted from the nail bed, and yellowish material builds under them. There may also be red spots in the nail as well as small spots of bleeding. Nail lesions often cause only cosmetic problems. They can, however, be painful when severe. Although about 40% of patients with psoriasis without psoriatic arthritis have nail lesions, nail involvement is much more frequent in patients with psoriatic arthritis where almost four out of five patients have nail lesions. Thus nail lesions are the only clinical feature that distinguishes patients with psoriatic arthritis from those with uncomplicated psoriasis. The nail bed is closely linked to the distal interphalangeal joint—the joint at the end of the fingers and toes. Severe involvement of the nail is associated with arthritis of these joints.

Extra-articular involvement

Apart from the involvement of the skin, nails, and joints, people with psoriatic arthritis also have involvement of other important organs. Eye involvement is not infrequent. Inflammation of the membrane covering the eye (conjunctiva), termed conjunctivitis, can lead to redness, eye discharge, and itching. It usually does not affect vision. More serious involvement of the eye can cause inflammation of the uvea, termed uveitis. Uveitis causes redness, pain, and blurred vision, and if untreated can lead to loss of vision. People with psoriatic arthritis also frequently complain of mouth sores due to inflammation of the mucosal surface of the mouth. Inflammation of the urethra can cause pain and burning while urinating. Inflammation of mucosal surfaces of the bowel can cause inflammatory bowel disease. Bowel involvement resembles

Crohn's disease and/or ulcerative colitis and can cause abdominal pain, loose stools, and bleeding. Severe inflammatory bowel disease can be life-threatening as it can cause rupture of the bowel, severe bleeding, and loss of bowel function.

Fatigue

Patients with psoriatic arthritis often complain of fatigue. It may be defined as an overwhelming, sustained sense of exhaustion and reduced capacity for physical and mental work. Fatigue is an important symptom in patients with chronic diseases, such as rheumatoid arthritis, systemic lupus erythematosus, and chronic liver disease. About 45% of patients with psoriatic arthritis report fatigue on clinical evaluation. When measured, using questionnaires, patients consistently score higher on fatigue scores than healthy controls. Changes in fatigue reflect changes in clinical disease activity in psoriatic arthritis. The level of fatigue as measured by questionnaires correlates with the degree of inflammation as measured by the actively inflamed joint count (number of swollen and/or tender joints), but not with the number of clinically damaged joints. Fatigue improves with effective treatment.

Physical function

Arthritis affects the ability of the affected individual to undertake day to day activities, be it avocational, vocational, or self-care activities. The degree to which arthritis affects daily activities depends on disease activity, extent of involvement, and the amount of damage. In patients with psoriatic arthritis, this is compounded by the presence of skin psoriasis. Physical functioning is measured using questionnaires, the most widely used one being the Health Assessment Questionnaire (HAQ). We have shown that disease activity as measured by the number of actively inflamed joints, and the number of clinically deformed joints, is a predictor of reduced physical function measured using the HAQ.

Health-related quality of life

Patients with psoriatic arthritis experience poor health-related quality of life compared with the general population. Quality of life is measured using questionnaires, the most commonly used being the Medical Outcomes Study 36-item Short Form health survey (SF-36). Using SF-36, we have shown that patients have poor physical functioning, increased pain, role limitations, and general health perception. It is well known that psoriasis alone contributes significantly to poor quality of life. In patients with psoriatic arthritis, this is compounded by the presence of inflammatory arthritis.

Laboratory investigations

Laboratory tests are usually done at diagnosis and periodically thereafter. However, there is to date no diagnostic test. The **acute phase reactants** (erythrocyte sedimentation rate (ESR) and C-reactive protein (CRP)) are often normal. These are raised in less than 50% of people with psoriatic arthritis. Rheumatoid factor is usually negative. The test for the HLA-B27 gene is usually not done, but is positive in 20% of patients with psoriatic arthritis. Radiological investigations (X-ray, ultrasonography, and magnetic resonance imaging (MRI)) can provide important clues to diagnosis and to the extent of inflammation and damage. However, only the presence of **periostitis** and new bone formation near joint margins may be considered reasonably specific to psoriatic arthritis. Although these tests are not by themselves diagnostic, they help in ruling out other conditions that may mimic psoriatic arthritis. Tests of the blood count, and liver and kidney functions are often obtained to monitor side effects of drug therapy.

A test that is often used is the aspiration and evaluation of synovial fluid. This test is important, especially when only a few joints are involved. Fluid is usually aspirated in the clinic, and sent immediately to the laboratory for examination. Aspirated joint fluid is usually inflammatory in nature in that the fluid is opaque, easily flows from the syringe into a container and has high white cell count. The fluid is usually clear of infection. Aspiration and laboratory analysis of joint fluid helps to rule out other arthritis conditions, since there are no diagnostic markers in the synovial fluid.

Synovial biopsy may be done, especially if there is destructive arthritis confined to one joint, to rule out infectious causes. Thus, it is often done to exclude other causes of arthritis. If a biopsy happens to be obtained from a patient with psoriatic arthritis, there are some characteristic features. There is increased thickness of the synovial membrane, a greatly increased number of blood vessels, and infiltration by **neutrophils** and **macrophages**. Pathologists often note that the features are similar to those of other spondyloarthritides and are different from rheumatoid arthritis.

Co-morbidities

Patients with psoriatic arthritis are at a higher risk of having **ischaemic heart disease** when compared to the general population. It is now well known that inflammation drives atherosclerosis, and people with inflammatory diseases such as rheumatoid arthritis and lupus have a higher risk of having future ischaemic heart disease. People with psoriatic arthritis, however, are not at an increased risk of having cancer. When compared with the general population, the risks are similar.

Mortality in psoriatic arthritis

Psoriatic arthritis has a significant effect on life span. Patients with psoriatic arthritis have an increased risk of mortality when compared with the general population. Those with a higher degree of inflammation, measured by the number of swollen and/or tender joints and blood tests of inflammation, are at increased risk of death. Overall, having psoriatic arthritis decreases one's life span by about 3 years.

Thus, psoriatic arthritis not only involves the joints and skin but can involve a number of body structures. Patients are at higher risk of death when compared with the general population, most commonly from heart disease.

6

Radiological features of psoriatic arthritis

> **→ Key points**
>
> ◆ Different imaging modalities may be used to detect inflammation and damage in psoriatic arthritis
>
> ◆ There are specific radiological features of peripheral joints
>
> ◆ There are specific radiological features of the spine

Imaging is an important tool in the assessment of patients with psoriatic arthritis. Imaging complements clinical assessment and helps in confirming the diagnosis as well as in determining the severity of psoriatic arthritis. The various modalities used in assessment of psoriatic arthritis include radiology (X-rays), ultrasound, computed tomography scan (CT scan), magnetic resonance imaging (MRI), and bone scan. The characteristic features of psoriatic arthritis seen with these radiological techniques are described here.

Plain radiographs (X-rays)

X-rays are the mainstay in the radiological assessment of psoriatic arthritis. X-rays are relatively cheap, easily available, and can be read by most physicians. Once psoriatic arthritis is suspected clinically, X-ray assessment of the hands, feet, pelvis, spine, and other affected joints is done to look for changes suggestive of psoriatic arthritis. Therefore, X-rays are used to help make the diagnosis of psoriatic arthritis. X-rays are also used to assess disease severity, as well as to follow disease progression. It should be noted, however, that X-ray changes generally reflect damage to the joints rather than acute inflammation.

In early disease, X-rays of the hands and feet show soft tissue swelling around the joints involved. If dactylitis is present, soft tissue swelling will involve the whole finger or toe. In more severe or long-standing disease, 'erosions' develop near the joint margin. Erosions are sites where the bone has been 'eaten away' by the inflamed synovial membrane. Erosions are markers of disease severity. Erosions may also be present slightly away from the joint margin, in contrast to rheumatoid arthritis where the erosions are very close to the joint margin. In psoriatic arthritis, erosions are often accompanied by 'new bone' formation. In fact the combination of erosions and new bone formation at joint margins is characteristic of psoriatic arthritis (Figs 6.1–3).

Changes seen on X-rays are often progressive. Early changes include soft tissue swelling without bone abnormalities. This is followed by erosions near joint margins, but no decrease in joint space—the space between the two ends of bones in the joint that reflects the thickness of cartilage. Progressive damage leads to an increase in the size and number of erosions as well as a decrease in joint space due to progressive breakdown of cartilage and bone. Ultimately, the joint is destroyed completely—either total joint lysis and the so-called 'pencil-in-cup' change or complete bony bridging through the joint termed ankylosis, essentially changing the two bones that make the joint into a single bone (Figs 6.4 and 6.5, p. 50).

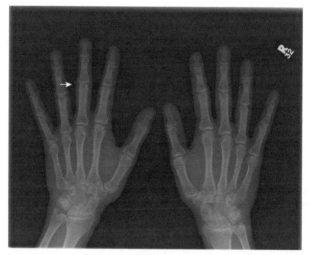

Figure 6.1 Early psoriatic arthritis—soft tissue swelling at the left third proximal interphalangeal joint in psoriatic arthritis.

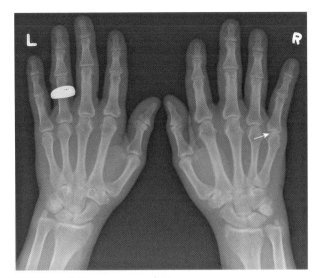

Figure 6.2 Erosive arthritis in psoriatic arthritis.

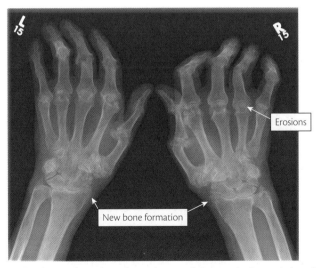

Figure 6.3 Erosions and new bone formation near joint margins in psoriatic arthritis.

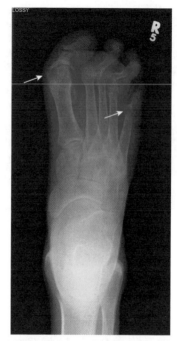

Figure 6.4 Pencil-in-cup change in the first metatarsophalangeal joint in psoriatic arthritis.

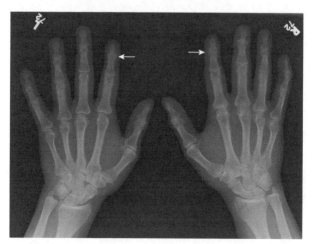

Figure 6.5 Complete fusion (ankylosis) of the bilateral second distal interphalangeal joint in psoriatic arthritis.

X-rays of the pelvis often show changes at the joints between the sacrum and the iliac bones deep inside the pelvis called the sacroiliac joints. These changes reflect the presence of sacroiliitis, or inflammation in the sacroiliac joints. The earliest notable changes include widening of the joint space, which is often difficult to appreciate. Subsequently, erosions develop, followed by increased whitening of the bone close to the joint (sclerosis), and subsequent bony bridging across the joints. Progressive sacroiliitis leads to complete fusion of the joint. Changes at the sacroiliac joints sometimes occur without clinical symptoms. Therefore, X-rays of the pelvis help in detecting its presence (Figs 6.6 and 6.7).

X-rays of the neck and the back often show changes that reflect consequences of inflammation at the **spinal joints**. These changes are best visualized on X-rays of the spine taken from the side (lateral view). The earliest changes include shiny upper and lower front corners of the individual vertebrae. This is followed by erosion of these corners. Erosions at the corners change the shape of the vertebrae and make them look more or less like a square. Therefore,

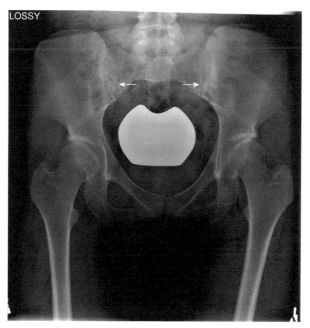

Figure 6.6 Erosions and sclerosis of both sacroiliac joints (Grade 2 sacroiliitis) in psoriatic arthritis.

51

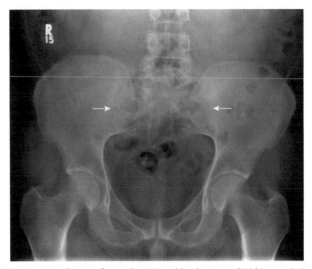

Figure 6.7 Complete fusion of sacroiliac joints (Grade 4 sacroiliitis) in psoriatic arthritis.

these changes are called 'squaring' of the vertebrae. This is followed by bone bridging, called 'marginal syndesmophytes', beginning from the ends of the vertebrae across the disc space. Complete bony bridging can occur. If most of the vertebrae are bridged, it is called 'bamboo' spine. These changes closely resemble the changes in ankylosing spondylitis. Often in psoriatic arthritis, however, the syndesmophytes can develop from sites away from the vertebral body. The presence of these 'non-marginal' syndesmophytes is characteristic of psoriatic arthritis. These syndesmophytes can also bridge vertebrae. The changes described can occur at any site—cervical and lumbar vertebrae are frequently involved. In the cervical spine, inflammation at the atlanto-axial joint, which is the joint between the first and second vertebrae, can lead to serious consequences. The second vertebra can get separated from the first vertebra and become dislocated. The dislocated second vertebra can then compress the spinal cord in the neck. Spinal cord compression in the neck can cause stiffness and weakness of the limbs and, sometimes, sudden death. X-rays of the neck taken from the side in full forward and backward bending help in diagnosing this condition (Figs 6.8 and 6.9, p. 53).

Ultrasound scans

An ultrasound scan can help greatly in the evaluation of both inflammation and damage in psoriatic arthritis. It can help to evaluate better the presence of

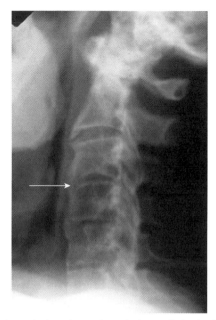

Figure 6.8 Classical marginal syndesmophytes in the cervical spine in psoriatic arthritis.

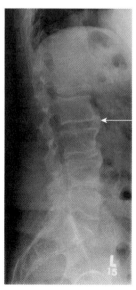

Figure 6.9 Non-marginal syndesmophytes in the lumbar spine in psoriatic arthritis.

swelling in the joints. Ultrasound also helps in evaluation of tendons and entheses (attachment of tendon into bone). Combined with Doppler evaluation, which can detect the amount of blood flow, ultrasound can help detect active inflammation in joints and entheses. This aspect of imaging cannot be detected by plain X-rays. Ultrasound can also detect erosions before they appear on X-rays, especially in hand joints. Since an ultrasound can be done at the bedside or in an outpatient clinic, it is a valuable tool in trained hands. It can also be used to guide injections into joints. Since ultrasound utilizes sound waves, there is no risk from exposure to radiation from ultrasound. Therefore, it can be done frequently and even in situations where exposure is to be avoided.

Magnetic resonance imaging

MRI scans have revolutionized the assessment of psoriatic arthritis, as they can detect both inflammation and damage. When a particular joint or region is suspected to be involved, MRI scans are valuable in providing details of the abnormalities. Tissues, such as synovial membrane, cartilage, tendons, and ligaments, are seen well on MRI. However, bone is not well visualized. MRI scans enhanced by injection of contrast material (gadolinium) can detect active inflammation. MRI can also show erosions in the bone even before they are seen on plain X-rays. Inflammation in the adjoining bone is also detected easily.

MRI scans are also very useful in detecting active inflammation in the spine. Inflammation and damage to sacroiliac joints can be detected, as can inflammation in the spinal vertebrae. Changes are usually evident well before any abnormality is visualized on X-rays. Thus MRI evaluation is crucial in the diagnosis of early disease, especially that affecting the spine. MRI scans also help in better evaluation of the cervical spine and to rule out dislocation of the first and second vertebrae and whether the spinal cord is involved. Cost and availability are the main limiting factors for widespread use of MRI. Contrast enhancement, which helps in detecting inflammation, adds to the cost. Usually, a single region is evaluated in one session. Moreover, patients with metal inside their body, for example those with joint replacements or those with devices such as pacemakers, cannot be evaluated using MRI. During the time when an MRI scan is carried out, the patient needs to lie still in a narrow enclosed chamber; people with claustrophobia might find it impossible.

Computed tomography scans

CT scans are most useful when joints or the spine need to be evaluated in detail, especially when an MRI cannot be done. CT scans also give a detailed view of the joints. Bones are viewed better than in MRIs. However, CT scans involve considerable exposure to radiation, and so frequent use is not recommended.

Bone scans

The techniques mentioned above help in detailed evaluation of a particular area that has been identified as having a problem on clinical evaluation. One way of imaging the entire skeletal system to identify areas affected by inflammation is by carrying out a whole body scan using radioactive isotopes. The isotope is injected into a vein and the uptake of the isotope at areas of inflammation is imaged using scanners. Such examination reveals areas of inflammation in joints and bone in patients with psoriatic arthritis. This type of imaging may be helpful to screen the entire skeletal system, to rule out the presence of inflammatory arthritis. Indeed, using bone scans, several investigators have shown that patients with psoriasis who are not thought to have active arthritis may indeed have subclinical inflammation in their joints or entheses.

Thus, nowadays a number of modalities are available to evaluate joints. Depending on the clinical question and stage of disease, the appropriate imaging modality is chosen to evaluate joints and the spine.

7

How is the diagnosis to psoriatic arthritis made?

> **Key points**
>
> - The diagnosis of psoriatic arthritis is dependent on:
>
>   - Clinical assessment
>
>   - Laboratory tests
>
>   - Radiological assessment
>
> - Standardized assessment is important in the evaluation of patients with psoriatic arthritis
>
> - The CASPAR criteria should help in correctly identifying patients with psoriatic arthritis

A number of arthritic conditions may occur in patients with psoriasis, and these must be differentiated from psoriatic arthritis. Since psoriasis is a common condition, occurring in 2–3% of the population, and rheumatoid arthritis, the most common form of inflammatory arthritis, may occur in 1% of the population, the co-occurrence of rheumatoid arthritis and psoriasis would be expected by chance alone in 1 in 10 000 people. Since rheumatoid arthritis, like psoriatic arthritis, is inflammatory in nature, the differentiation may be difficult. Osteoarthritis, which is the most common form of arthritis, occurs in about 5% of the population and it may co-exist with psoriasis. While osteoarthritis is not usually an inflammatory form of arthritis, it does affect the end joints of the fingers, a site commonly affected in patients with psoriatic arthritis, and therefore one needs to differentiate osteoarthritis from psoriatic arthritis. Psoriatic arthritis may sometimes be misdiagnosed as gout. Gout is a crystal-induced arthritis caused by uric acid deposition in the joints.

Some patients with psoriatic arthritis may present with a red hot swollen joint which may be considered to be gout, when in fact it may be psoriatic arthritis. Another set of conditions that require differentiation from psoriatic arthritis are the other members of the spondyloarthritis group.

 Myth

Psoriatic arthritis can be diagnosed from blood tests.

 Fact

Blood tests are not diagnostic, but help to rule out other arthritic conditions. The diagnosis is made from careful clinical, laboratory, and radiographic assessment.

Clinical features which help diagnose psoriatic arthritis

While several conditions must be differentiated from psoriatic arthritis, there are a number of clinical and radiological features which can help. The diagnosis of psoriatic arthritis is considered when a patient presents with inflammatory musculoskeletal disease. This may be in the form of arthritis, dactylitis, enthesitis, or spondylitis. The presence of skin psoriasis is an important clue, and this should be looked for carefully, especially in hidden regions such as the scalp, belly-button, below the breasts, or between the buttocks. Nails should be carefully inspected for changes of nail psoriasis as the evidence of psoriasis may be present in the nail only. Moreover, most patients with psoriatic arthritis have nail involvement compared with only about half of patients with psoriasis alone.

The next clue is the pattern of joints involved. Involvement of distal interphalangeal joints (end joints of the fingers and toes) is characteristic. While, as mentioned above, this is a feature of osteoarthritis, the latter is not usually an inflammatory condition. Patients will complain of pain but usually no swelling or morning stiffness, and the pain will be worse with activity rather than with rest.

The pattern of involvement in psoriatic arthritis is often asymmetric, that is the same joints are not involved on both sides of the body. This is not usually the case in rheumatoid arthritis, which tends to be very symmetric. A characteristic pattern of psoriatic arthritis is the 'ray' pattern—involvement of all joints in a particular finger or toe, as opposed to joints beside one another (Fig. 7.1). This is typical for psoriatic arthritis, and is not usually seen in either rheumatoid arthritis or osteoarthritis.

The presence of dactylitis is an important feature. It is a typical feature for psoriatic arthritis and is not seen in rheumatoid arthritis. The only other arthritis condition which may manifest with dactylitis is reactive arthritis, which is not associated with psoriasis.

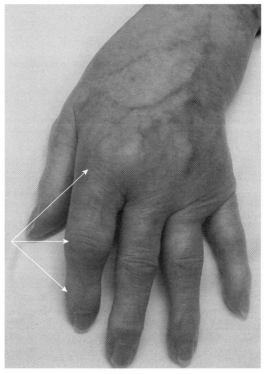

Figure 7.1 Involvement of the second metacarpophalangeal, proximal interphalangeal, and distal interphalangeal joints ('ray' involvement) in psoriatic arthritis.

Spinal involvement presenting as inflammatory neck or back pain with or without restriction of mobility is present in about half of the patients with psoriatic arthritis, especially in well established disease. It is not a feature of rheumatoid arthritis. The presence of spinal and peripheral arthritis makes the diagnosis of psoriatic arthritis very likely, and virtually rules out diseases such as rheumatoid arthritis.

The diagnosis of psoriatic arthritis may sometimes be made even in the absence of psoriasis. If the above characteristic features are present even without skin psoriasis, the diagnosis may be considered. The diagnosis is especially likely if there is a family history of psoriasis or psoriatic arthritis. The diagnosis may also be made if characteristic radiographic features such as 'pencil-in-cup' changes, bony ankylosis, new bone formation close to sites of erosions, and non-marginal syndesmophytes are present.

 Myth

The degree of inflammation in psoriatic arthritis is reflected in blood tests for inflammation.

 Fact

Blood tests for inflammation, such as erythrocyte sedimentation rate and C-reactive protein levels, are normal in up to 50% of patients with psoriatic arthritis. Therefore, joint counts (number of swollen and/or tender joints) are used to assess the degree of inflammation in peripheral joints.

Laboratory tests in psoriatic arthritis

Blood tests have only a minor role to play in making the diagnosis of psoriatic arthritis. Characteristically, rheumatoid factor test is negative, although a positive test does not rule out the diagnosis. Markers of inflammation in the blood such as an elevated erythrocyte sedimentation rate (ESR) or C-reactive protein (CRP) are present only in about half of the patients. However, these are markers of severity. Other tests usually done are routine tests such as blood counts, and liver and kidney function tests. Although these tests are not important in making a diagnosis, they give important information on the presence of co-morbid conditions and are important in monitoring treatment. If **synovial**

fluid can be aspirated from the joint, it can be tested to confirm inflammation and to rule out other causes of inflammation such as infection and crystals. **Synovial biopsies**, usually done using an **arthroscope**, show evidence of chronic inflammation, and are sometimes required to rule out chronic infection.

Imaging

Imaging has a crucial role in making a diagnosis. X-rays show evidence of involvement of joints, with changes ranging from soft tissue swelling to complete destruction. Features that help in making a correct diagnosis include erosions and new bone formation. X-rays also help in identifying arthritis in the spine. Plain X-rays show evidence of past damage, and can often be normal in early disease. In such a situation, other modalities of imaging such as Doppler ultrasound and, more importantly, MRI can help in identifying areas of inflammation and the presence of joint involvement and damage that is not visible on X-rays. Bone scans may help in identifying joints affected by inflammation. Thus, imaging plays an important role in making a diagnosis, especially when physical examination is equivocal.

Classification criteria for psoriatic arthritis—the CASPAR criteria

The development of the CASPAR criteria for the classification of psoriatic arthritis should facilitate the diagnosis of psoriatic arthritis. According to the CASPAR criteria, if a patient has inflammatory joint, spine, or entheseal disease, and they have psoriasis, and one of nail lesions, dactylitis, negative rheumatoid factor, or periosteal reaction on the X-rays, this will qualify the patients as having psoriatic arthritis. If the patient does not have psoriasis, but has a family history of psoriasis or a personal history of psoriasis and two of the other above-mentioned features, the patient could be classified as having psoriatic arthritis. Even in the absence of psoriasis, a patient with inflammatory musculoskeletal disease could be classified as having psoriatic arthritis if they have any three of the following features: dactylitis, nail lesions, negative rheumatoid factor, or periosteal reaction (Table 7.1, p. 62).

Thus, after a complete history and physical examination, and with information obtained from imaging and laboratory tests, a rheumatologist makes a diagnosis of psoriatic arthritis.

Table 7.1 CASPAR criteria for classification of psoriatic arthritis

Inflammatory musculoskeletal disease (joint, spine, or entheseal) with three or more of the following:

1. Evidence of psoriasis (one of a, b, or c)	a. Current psoriasis*	Psoriatic skin or scalp disease present today as judged by a dermatologist or
	b. Personal history of psoriasis	A history of psoriasis that may be obtained from patient, family doctor, dermatologist, or rheumatologist or
	c. Family history of psoriasis	A history of psoriasis in a first- or second-degree relative according to patient report
2. Psoriatic nail dystrophy		Typical psoriatic nail dystrophy including onycholysis, pitting, and hyperkeratosis observed on current physical examination
3. A negative test for rheumatoid factor		By any method except latex but preferably by ELISA or nephelometry, according to the local laboratory reference range
4. Dactylitis (either a or b)	a. Current dactylitis	Swelling of an entire digit
	b. History of dactylitis	Recorded by a rheumatologist
5. Radiological evidence of juxta-articular new bone formation		Ill-defined ossification near joint margins (but excluding osteophyte formation) on plain X-rays of hand or foot

*Current psoriasis scores 2; others 1.

ELISA = enzyme-linked immunosorbent assay.

Standardized assessment in psoriatic arthritis

Once the diagnosis is confirmed, disease manifestations have to be systematically assessed so that future change in disease can be determined, in particular to decide whether a specific treatment is working. Thus, the skin, nails, joints, dactylitis, entheses, and back are assessed in a standard way.

The extent and severity of psoriasis is usually rated using a scoring system called the psoriasis area and severity index (PASI). The amount of body surface area covered by psoriasis is recorded. The number of nails affected and, for a more objective rating, a nail psoriasis severity index is calculated. The number of tender and swollen joints is recorded as well as the number of joints with clinical damage. Dactylitis, if present, is recorded. The number of tender entheseal sites is counted. The extent of movement in the spine is recorded using a series of manoeuvres. The extent to which the lower spine can bend forward is measured using Schober's test. Bending sideways is assessed by measuring the range of movement between standing straight and fully bending to the side. Chest expansion and neck rotation are recorded. The subject is also asked to stand straight against a wall, and the presence and degree of forward stoop is recorded by measuring the distance between the wall and the back of the head. These factors are typically examined periodically in the same standard way, so that improvement or worsening can be measured objectively.

Similarly, X-rays and MRI can also be scored in a systematic way. With plain X-rays, the number of joints showing erosions and the degree of damage is recorded. The degree of sacroiliitis, the presence of squaring of vertebrae, and the presence and extent of syndesmophytes are recorded. Composite scores for peripheral arthritis and spinal changes are then recorded, higher scores indicating more damage. Similarly, MRI of the spine can be scored for the presence of inflammatory lesions using specialized scoring systems. Since MRI reflects active inflammation, higher scores indicate more active disease.

Patient-reported outcomes

Outcomes that are self-reported by patients are also important. These are usually measured using questionnaires. Questionnaires are used to measure pain, fatigue, physical function, and health-related quality of life. These questionnaires are given to patients periodically and this is ideally done just prior to the rheumatologist's assessment. The questionnaires include a visual analogue scale for pain, FACIT-fatigue scale for fatigue, HAQ for physical function, and SF-36 for quality of life.

Thus, after a comprehensive clinical and radiological evaluation, your rheumatologist makes a diagnosis and rates the degree of disease activity. Future evaluations and scores are then compared with the scores obtained initially to help make treatment decisions.

8

Functional and emotional impact

⮕ Key points

◆ Quality of life and function are important components of the impact of the psoriasis and psoriatic arthritis on the patients affected by these conditions

◆ There are both generic and disease-specific instruments to measure the effect on quality of life. These have been tested in patients with psoriatic arthritis and have shown impairment which improves with appropriate therapy

◆ Physical function is reduced among patients with psoriatic arthritis, but improves with appropriate medications which control disease activity

◆ Psoriasis and psoriatic arthritis affect the emotional state of patients. These need to be evaluated and treated

◆ Fatigue is an important issue for patients with psoriatic arthritis. It can be measured by a validated instrument and shows a correlation with disease activity and improvement with appropriate therapy

◆ A new concept to evaluate the effect of disease on all facets of a person's life has been developed, termed participation. Participation is currently being investigated in psoriasis and psoriatic arthritis

Chronic disease is bound to exert an effect on an individual's quality of life and function. Psoriatic arthritis is no exception. Psoriasis is a chronic relapsing condition, which at times may be disfiguring, while psoriatic arthritis is a chronic often deforming and progressive inflammatory arthritis.

Patients with psoriatic arthritis are thus doubly affected, first by their chronic skin condition, the psoriasis, and secondly by their chronic, often debilitating arthritis. Therefore, there is an important functional and emotional impact of psoriatic arthritis. Indeed, a number of studies in the past several years have demonstrated the impact of their condition on the physical, social, and emotional well-being of patients with psoriasis and psoriatic arthritis.

Physical effects

The physical effect of psoriasis can be clearly seen. Psoriasis presents with red scaly lesions. In some patients, these may be limited to the scalp or other areas that are not obviously visible, while in other patients the lesions may be on the face, hands, arms, and legs, where they are very obvious. Moreover, the psoriatic lesions may be very itchy, a fact which contributes to the discomfort felt by the patient. While the arthritis may not be as painful as other forms of arthritis, it certainly is associated with pain and swelling and can lead to joint deformities, which are very obvious, particularly if these changes are accompanied by psoriatic skin lesions. These physical features may lead to a distorted perception of self-image by the affected individual. Indeed, in the 2001 National Psoriasis Foundation Survey, 75% of the responders reported feeling unattractive. Of the patients who responded to the survey, 79% believed that their psoriasis had a major impact on their lives. A European study found that 60% of the patients had significant problems related to their psoriasis.

Psychological effects

The above-noted physical features affect the patients' psychological well-being as well. Depression has been reported to be increased among patients with psoriasis compared with the general population. Depression may be associated with more severe symptoms of psoriasis. Fifty-four per cent of the responders to the National Psoriasis Foundation Survey reported feeling depressed because of their psoriasis. In addition, 81% were embarrassed when others viewed their psoriasis. Patients with psoriasis also describe feelings of helplessness and frustration about their disease. Moreover, 57% of responders reported that their psoriasis was considered contagious by others and confused with other conditions. This, of course, is another source of frustration for the patients affected by this disease, particularly when using services such as a barber and hairdresser, or public swimming pools.

Although similar studies have not been performed specifically among patients with psoriatic arthritis, it is clear that these patients are going to feel these frustrations even more, since not only do they have the psoriasis to deal with, but they also have the arthritis which adds to the physical issues and further inability to carry out daily activities.

Effect on quality of life

The majority of the responders to the National Psoriasis Foundation Survey reported that the psoriasis had an impact on their lives. Over the past two decades there has been a growing science of assessment and measurement of the effect of a disease on patient quality of life and function. Several instruments have been developed which can not only determine whether there is impaired quality of life or function, but can also quantitate the degree of impairment. Some of these measures are generic; they are not specific to a particular disease and they work in many diseases and allow for comparisons between different conditions. Others are disease specific, designed for certain diseases. While these disease-specific questionnaires measure the quality of life in patients with a particular disease, they are specific to that disease and do not allow comparison with other conditions.

The most commonly used generic quality of life instrument is the Medical Outcome Survey Short Form 36 (SF-36). This is a 36-item questionnaire which covers both physical and mental health aspects in eight domains on a 0–100 scale. Higher numbers reflect better quality of life. Healthy individuals usually score above 80 on these domains. Patients with psoriasis and psoriatic arthritis score much lower in each of these domains than the general population, confirming that their quality of life is worse than that of healthy individuals. The SF-36 is useful in that its scores may be used to compare people suffering from a variety of conditions. Using this scale, it has been possible to demonstrate that patients with psoriasis rate their quality of life as poorly as patients with diabetes and worse than those with cancer, heart attacks, or high blood pressure. Using the same tool, patients with psoriatic arthritis report their quality of life to be much lower than that of the general population. In addition to analysing the eight individual domains of the SF-36, it is possible to combine the domains into a physical function summary and a mental function summary. Using these two summary scores, values close to 60 are obtained from healthy individuals. Both of these components have been shown to be much lower in patients with psoriasis and psoriatic arthritis (with scores just above 40) compared with the general population and patients with other chronic conditions (with scores ranging from 43 to 53). The SF-36 has been used in clinical trials and it was shown that patients who respond to treatment also improved their SF-36 scores.

Some investigators have argued that the generic quality of life instrument does not capture all of the issues that are important to patients with psoriasis and psoriatic arthritis, and have developed disease-specific instruments. The dermatology life quality index (DLQI) is a questionnaire specifically developed for patients suffering from skin conditions. The DLQI consists of 10 items, with a total possible score of 30, with higher scores reflecting lower quality of life. Although developed specifically for dermatology, the 10 items span a variety of topics including symptoms, feelings, daily activities, work/school, relationships, and treatment. The DLQI demonstrated the reduced quality of life of patients with psoriasis compared with healthy controls. The DLQI was sensitive to change in clinical trials, showing that patients who received active drugs had a greater reduction in DLQI scores (improvement) than those receiving placebo. The DLQI has been the most commonly studied instrument of quality of life in randomized controlled trials of new drugs in psoriasis and psoriatic arthritis.

Other disease-specific instruments to assess quality of life have been developed. These include the psoriasis quality of life instrument and the psoriatic arthritis quality of life instrument both developed in the UK. Both instruments show good properties but have not yet been tested in clinical trials, thus their responsiveness is unknown.

Function in psoriasis and psoriatic arthritis

The instrument most commonly used to measure function in psoriatic arthritis is the Health Assessment Questionnaire (HAQ). While it was first developed for assessing patients with rheumatoid arthritis, it proved useful in patients with psoriatic arthritis as well. The HAQ assesses physical function over the previous week and consists of 20 questions that cover eight categories of daily living: dressing and grooming, arising, eating, walking, hygiene, reach, grip, and activities including errands and chores. The scores of the eight categories are averaged to obtain an overall score on a scale from 0 reflecting no disability to 3 reflecting severe disability. Patients with psoriatic arthritis demonstrate higher HAQ scores (meaning more disability) that the general population, but on average their scores are not as high as those of patients with rheumatoid arthritis. The HAQ scores correlated with features of disease activity and damage in patients with psoriatic arthritis. Among patients with psoriatic arthritis included in recent randomized controlled trials, the HAQ scores were quite high, suggesting moderate disability. These scores improved significantly in patients treated with active drugs compared with placebo. The new biological agents have clearly proven their ability to improve the HAQ scores. It is not clear whether the HAQ is useful in patients with psoriasis who do not have arthritis.

A HAQ score which includes questions on psoriasis was also developed and tested, but provided the same results as the HAQ without the psoriasis questions in patients with psoriatic arthritis.

Assessment of fatigue

Fatigue is an important symptom in patients with psoriatic arthritis, although it is not clear whether it is important in patients suffering from skin lesions only. Fatigue has been assessed by asking patients whether they feel that fatigue interferes with their activities of daily living, or by using specific instruments developed to quantify fatigue. Two such instruments have been used in psoriatic arthritis. The Fatigue Severity Scale (FSS) was originally developed for assessing patients with **multiple sclerosis** and systemic lupus erythematosus. It consists of nine questions related to fatigue, each scored between 0—meaning no effect at all—and 10—meaning completely affected by fatigue. This instrument was validated in patients with psoriatic arthritis and found to be reliable and sensitive to change. Changes in fatigue measured by the FSS were found to correlate with changes in disease activity, suggesting that the fatigue was in some way related to the inflammatory process itself.

Another measure of fatigue developed initially for the assessment of cancer patients is called the Functional Assessment of Chronic Illness Therapy (FACIT)-fatigue score. Responses to the 13 items on the FACIT-fatigue questionnaire are each measured on a 4-point scale, with the total score ranging from 0 to 52. High scores represent less fatigue. The FACIT-fatigue scale has been validated in the general population, in patients with cancer, rheumatoid arthritis, and recently in psoriatic arthritis. The FACIT-fatigue scale correlated with the FSS, as well as with the presence of overwhelming fatigue as reported by the patient. In addition, the FACIT-fatigue scale correlated with the number of actively inflamed joints. Improvement in FACIT-fatigue scores correlated with in recent drug trials response.

Participation

The instruments described above for the assessment of quality of life and function focus specifically on the ability of individuals to perform tasks that are necessary for daily living. However, they do not take into account the actual efficiency of performing those tasks, nor do they include leisure and pleasure activities. Through the World Health Organization (WHO), new instruments are being developed in which all aspects of the effects of disease on patients' lives have been addressed. There is a new concept of participation, the ability of an individual to participate in all lives events. Psoriatic arthritis is one of the conditions for which participation instruments are being developed. Through the efforts of GRAPPA (Group for Research and Assessment of Psoriasis and Psoriatic Arthritis), several collaborative studies have begun in which patients and physicians have participated in developing the items that need to be assessed. In addition, a number of centres have participated in a study in which participation instruments have been completed by patients with psoriatic arthritis. These studies are currently being analysed, and the results should be available within the next year.

Summary

It is clear that quality of life and function are important components of the impact of psoriasis and psoriatic arthritis on the patients affected by these conditions. As patients with psoriasis and psoriatic arthritis are being treated, it is important that both the patient and the physician pay attention to the effect of the disease, in addition to the documentation of the extent and severity of the skin and joint manifestations.

It will be important to use therapeutic modalities which not only work on the physical aspect of the disease but also improve the effect on the patient, as measured by the fatigue, quality of life, and function.

9

Non-drug therapy

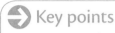 **Key points**

◆ Physical and occupational therapy are important in the management of psoriatic arthritis

◆ They help limit the disability due to joint disease and improve the overall quality of life for the patients

As with all chronic rheumatic conditions, treatment of psoriatic arthritis involves care by a multidisciplinary team. Although pharmacotherapy with drugs is the cornerstone of treatment of inflammatory arthritis such as psoriatic arthritis, non-drug therapy also plays a valuable role. Comprehensive care of a patient with psoriatic arthritis requires integrated drug and non-drug therapies and educational intervention. Non-drug therapy chiefly includes education, and physical and occupational therapy.

Education

It is most important for patients to be educated regarding their condition. Nowadays it is quite easy for patients to gain knowledge through the Internet. However, some information gained from the Internet is not necessarily accurate. Therefore, much time is spent educating patients as to the nature of inflammatory arthritis, the relationship between the skin and joint disease, as well as the other features of the disease and the co-morbidities which may occur in patients with psoriatic arthritis. This book is designed specifically for patient education.

Similar approaches have been taken at other centres. There are often public lectures dealing with inflammatory arthritis and, in many centres where experts in psoriatic arthritis are present, there are specific lectures on psoriatic arthritis. Many dermatologists provide educational lectures on psoriasis and its associated arthritis.

An educated patient will appreciate the need for early therapy, as well as the role of the non-drug interventions, in the management of psoriatic arthritis.

Physical therapy

Benefits of low impact exercises are seen across all age groups in patients with and without arthritis, and patients with psoriatic arthritis are no exception. More specific exercise regimens are of help to patients. Although exercise programmes specific to psoriatic arthritis have not been developed, since psoriatic arthritis can affect both the peripheral arthritis and the spine, exercise programmes developed for rheumatoid arthritis and ankylosing spondylitis are recommended to patients with psoriatic arthritis.

When psoriatic arthritis is active, and the patient has a number of swollen and painful joints, physical therapy may not be feasible. In this situation, rest and drug treatment to relieve pain and inflammation should be instituted. As soon as symptoms improve, physical therapy should commence. Measures to relieve symptoms would depend on the area of the musculoskeletal system that is primarily involved—peripheral or axial.

Physical therapy includes that provided within the physical therapy department and exercise regimes at the patient's own home. Initially the patients may benefit from therapy provided at a physical therapy department but, once they have mastered the exercises, it would be more feasible and less expensive to continue with the exercises at home, and incorporate these exercises into the daily routine of life.

Initially, physical therapists would assess the physical and functional status and evaluate the joints, heart, and lungs. They would teach methods for pain relief, and improvement in mobility, balance, and gait, especially in the elderly. Physiotherapists would also teach exercises to improve flexibility, muscle strength, and endurance. Because of pain and immobility, people with active arthritis may develop cardiovascular deconditioning, muscle weakness, and decreased endurance. This greatly affects their physical function. Regular conditioning exercises improve both function and quality of life. The major forms of exercise that are recommended for patients with psoriatic arthritis include flexibility and range of motion exercises, muscle conditioning, and aerobic exercises.

Range of motion exercises

Psoriatic arthritis, being an inflammatory arthritis, results in joint damage and loss of motion at the peripheral joints as well as the spine. Therefore, regular range of motion exercises are important in patients with psoriatic arthritis to maintain joint function and flexibility in the peripheral joints and the spine. Range of motion exercises also help decrease morning stiffness. Patients with psoriatic arthritis are advised to continue such exercises as part of their daily routine.

Muscle conditioning exercises

Muscle strengthening exercises improve strength, decrease pain, and improve function. Muscle strengthening exercises may be of different intensities. These exercises may range from low intensity exercises done at home, through moderate intensity training of specific muscle groups, to high intensity training under supervision. The nature and intensity would have to be individualized and planned in consultation with a physical therapist as this would depend on various factors including the patient's age, the joints involved, co-morbidities, and the treatment goal. Some patients seek advice from personal trainers. While such programmes may be appropriate for individuals who are no longer suffering from active inflammation, it is important to check with a health professional before embarking on active training exercises.

In general, therapy is initiated under supervision of a physical therapist with expertise in the management of arthritic conditions who understands the principles of joint protection and graded resistance exercise training. Joints with significant damage, e.g. instability or malalignment, have to be protected. Patients with spinal involvement have pain, restriction of movement, and, subsequently, spinal deformities. These patients benefit from physical therapy approaches used in the management of ankylosing spondylitis. Correction of bad posture and extension exercises for the back are important in preventing spinal deformities and maintaining function. Deep breathing exercises improve chest expansion. In patients with psoriatic arthritis, restriction of neck movement is particularly bothersome. Regular range of motion exercises are important in maintaining neck mobility. After a few weeks of education and supervision, patients are usually in a position to continue the therapy at home. Periodic reinforcement and motivation improves long-term outcome.

Aerobic exercises

Aerobic exercises help improve function, cardiovascular fitness, and quality of life. This class of exercises includes activities such as walking, cycling, and aerobic dance and pool routines. Most patients can safely participate in these activities without worsening joint damage. However, the presence of severe skin psoriasis may prevent patients from taking part in these activities, especially swimming pool routines, in a group. Motivation to continue these activities is crucial. Community programmes and patient self-help groups, if available, go a long way in motivating patients to maintain the exercise programme.

Other modalities of physical therapy

Other methods of physical therapy include use of physical modalities such as heat, cold, and ultrasound. Heat is applied superficially using hot packs, paraffin, or hydrotherapy, or as deep heat using diathermy or ultrasound. Heat application relieves pain, decreases muscle spasm, promotes relaxation, and improves function in peripheral joints and the spine. In patients with enthesitis and tendonitis, local treatment using ultrasound helps in reducing pain and inflammation. Cold application with cold packs or with ice may improve symptoms especially when applied to very inflamed joints. Some patients also get relief of pain from transcutaneous electrical nerve stimulation (TENS). TENS may decrease inflammation. The above methods of physical therapy may be taught to patients and, once proven to be effective, used at home along with other modalities of treatment.

Occupational therapy

Joint protection and energy conservation are important in the management of chronic arthritic conditions. These measures reduce pain, protect joints from further damage, and improve function and quality of life. Early referral to an occupational therapist is recommended. Patients are taught how to modify their routine at home and work so as to conserve energy. Assistive devices are used to protect joints. The home and work environment is modified towards these goals.

Hand function may be significantly compromised in patients with psoriatic arthritis. Splinting of the wrists and hands helps immobilization and provides support. This helps in decreasing inflammation, supports function, and reduces formation of deformities. Splints may be functional splints used to help function, corrective splints to correct deformities, or resting splints that are worn during rest, especially at night.

Patients with psoriatic arthritis have frequent foot and heel pain due to plantar fasciitis and Achilles tendonitis. Midfoot and forefoot joints are also frequently inflamed. Foot orthoses, either custom made or otherwise, help relieve symptoms in conjunction with other measures. A number of types of orthoses, heel pads, and lifts help relieve pain and improve gait. Rigid orthoses are usually custom made and are used to prevent unnecessary motion and to maintain alignment. Semi-rigid orthoses are used to provide support and redistribute force, and are usually available in pharmacies. If significant deformities are present, a trained orthotist can design the most useful orthotic device. In patients with mild foot disease, athletic shoes and shock-absorbing insoles provide adequate pain relief. Proper use of a walking stick helps in relief of pain associated with hip movement in patients with hip disease.

Summary

The comprehensive management of patients with psoriatic arthritis involves early referral to physical and occupational therapists, in conjunction with drug therapy. Energy conservation, joint protection, range of motion exercises, and local treatment of problem sites such as entheses and tendons help relieve pain, improve functions, and increase overall quality of life.

10

Drug therapy

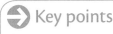
Key points

- Pharmacotherapy is key to the management of psoriatic arthritis

- NSAIDs are used to treat mild disease and for symptom relief

- DMARDs are the first line of management, although they have not been shown to be very effective

- Biological agents, especially anti-TNF agents, are effective in relieving symptoms, improving function, and preventing joint damage

Pharmacotherapy or drug therapy is the cornerstone of management of psoriatic arthritis. Drug therapy depends on the severity and stage of the arthritis and the severity of skin disease. Patients should ideally be under the care of a team of health professionals comprising rheumatologists, dermatologists, physiotherapists, and occupational therapists. However, if the primary problem is skin disease and the arthritis is mild, the subject may be managed by a dermatologist after a complete assessment by a rheumatologist. Periodic assessment by a rheumatologist in such cases would be ideal. On the other hand, if the primary problem is joint disease, the rheumatologist should primarily manage the patient, with the dermatologist confirming the diagnosis of psoriasis and providing input if skin disease remains poorly controlled.

Drug therapy for psoriatic arthritis may be classified into

1. Symptom-modifying therapy

2. Therapy with 'disease-modifying' anti-rheumatic drugs (DMARDs)

3. Therapy with biological agents

Symptom-modifying therapy

Non-steroidal anti-inflammatory drugs (NSAIDs)

NSAIDs are useful in the treatment of psoriatic arthritis and give relief of symptoms such as pain and stiffness. However, NSAIDs do not prevent disease progression, and may worsen skin lesions. They may be used as sole therapy in treating mild psoriatic arthritis and for symptomatic management of pain, inflammatory swelling, and morning stiffness. With the recent reports of increased risk of heart attacks and stroke with long-term use of the newer COX-2 (cyclo-oxygenase-2) inhibitors, the use of non-selective NSAIDs such as naproxen, ibuprofen, diclofenac, indomethacin, or aspirin (with or without misoprostol/H_2-blockers/proton pump inhibitors) would be preferable. If symptoms persist after adequate trial with two different NSAIDs, disease-modifying anti-rheumatic drug (DMARD) use should be considered.

 Myth

Treatment with corticosteroids is effective in psoriatic arthritis.

 Fact

Systemic corticosteroids have not been shown to be effective, although intra-articular injections help relieve symptoms. Corticosteroids may worsen psoriasis, especially when the dose is being tapered. Long-term steroid therapy has many well-recognized adverse effects.

Corticosteroids

Corticosteroid therapy may be in the form of **intra-articular injections** or injections of corticosteroids (triamcinolone, methylprednisolone) into the joints either at the bedside in the clinic or under ultrasound guidance. Corticosteroids are often used for rapid relief of symptoms in cases where only one or a few joints are affected. In such cases the disease may be controlled with one or a few injections. Corticosteroids may also be injected into inflamed tendon sheaths to relieve pain and swelling associated with tendonitis. Corticosteroids taken orally are used occasionally for symptom relief when there is polyarthritis or when there is inadequate response to NSAIDs. However, corticosteroids need to be used with extreme caution with a slow decrease in dose, since psoriasis worsens in many instances and could occasionally evolve into more severe forms such as pustular psoriasis. Treatment with oral corticosteroids is usually resorted to as short-term therapy, until other longer acting drugs take effect. Long-term corticosteroid therapy is associated with significant toxicity such as high blood pressure, cataracts, weight gain, stretch marks on the skin, diabetes, osteoporosis, and **avascular necrosis of bone**, especially in the hips.

Disease-modifying drug therapy

In patients with persistently active disease despite treatment with NSAIDs and/or joint injections, or in those with evidence of damage on X-rays in the form of erosions, a class of drugs called disease-modifying anti-rheumatic drugs (DMARDs) is usually used as the first line of treatment. In order that they control disease well, they should be used early in the disease course. Most drugs belonging to this class work for both the joints and the skin. The important DMARDs are reviewed here.

Methotrexate

Methotrexate is the most widely used DMARD in psoriatic arthritis. There are, however, only two controlled trials of its use in psoriatic arthritis. One showed efficacy but the methotrexate was given intravenously and caused significant toxicity. The other used oral methotrexate but did not show significant improvement. The dose of methotrexate used in that trial was too low, and the number of patients too small to demonstrate efficacy. Uncontrolled studies have demonstrated good results with use of methotrexate in psoriatic arthritis; however, methotrexate has not been shown to reduce progression in erosions on radiographs.

Although methotrexate is also used in high doses in the treatment of cancer, as a DMARD it is typically used in low doses. Over the last decade, methotrexate has been used typically in doses ranging from 15 to 25 mg once a week. It is typically taken orally, although it is preferably given by **subcutaneous injections** whenever doses higher than 15 or 17.5 mg/week are required.

However, methotrexate has the potential to cause significant adverse events. Many patients complain of nausea and fatigue, especially for a few days after methotrexate is taken. More serious adverse events include liver toxicity and decrease in blood counts. Alcohol consumption is strictly prohibited when one is on methotrexate as it can increase the risk of both short- and long-term liver toxicity, leading to cirrhosis of the liver. The risk of liver toxicity is higher in people who continue to consume methotrexate, are diabetic, and overweight. Poor renal function also increases the risk of adverse effects of methotrexate. Therefore, blood tests to test for liver functions and blood counts have to be done at monthly intervals to detect early toxicity. Some physicians, especially dermatologists, recommend regular liver biopsy to look for evidence of liver toxicity. We recommend liver biopsies only if liver function tests are persistently abnormal even after therapy with methotrexate is discontinued. Methotrexate is **teratogenic** and is therefore contraindicated in women with child-bearing potential.

Sulfasalazine

Although sulfasalazine is commonly used in the treatment of psoriatic arthritis, its efficacy in this condition is modest. There are a few controlled trials of sulfasalazine in psoriatic arthritis. In these trials, the number of patients treated was small and there was a small improvement in symptoms and signs of psoriatic arthritis. Although sulfasalazine may improve symptoms, it does not prevent progression of radiographic damage. It is also associated with significant toxicity—sulfa allergy can be life threatening. Blood counts and liver function have to be monitored. Some patients also develop severe headaches after taking the drug.

Antimalarials

Chloroquine has been used in the treatment of psoriatic arthritis, although exacerbation of psoriasis may occur. However, it has not been shown to be effective in reducing symptoms and signs or preventing radiographic progression. Chloroquine is also not without toxicity. Significant eye (retinal) damage can occur, and the eyes have to be monitored by an ophthalmologist regularly, to detect early toxicity so that the drug treatment is stopped and damage reversed. Hydroxychloroquine is similar in action to chloroquine but has less eye toxicity. Its efficacy in psoriatic arthritis is unknown.

Cyclosporin A

Cyclosporin A is effective in controlling psoriasis. It has been compared with other DMARDs and was shown to be better in controlling pain compared with sulfasalazine when added to NSAIDs and low dose corticosteroids. When compared with methotrexate, it was found to be equally efficacious, but more patients stopped cyclosporin A due to adverse events. In patients showing an incomplete response to methotrexate, addition of cyclosporin A to methotrexate led to improvement in swollen joints and PASI score, but no improvement was shown in pain or physical function. Thus, cyclosporin A may have a role in patients with partial response to methotrexate as an add-on treatment.

However, cyclosporin A is associated with significant adverse events. Blood pressure is often elevated and kidney function is affected. Since it is an **immunosuppressant**, patients on cyclosporin A are at higher risk of serious infections. Liver functions also have to be monitored.

Azathioprine

Although occasionally used in the treatment of psoriatic arthritis, there is no evidence that azathioprine improves symptoms or prevents disease progression.

Leflunomide

Leflunomide was recently shown to be an effective treatment of psoriatic arthritis in a multicentre controlled trial comparing it with **placebo**. The arthritis improved and there was improvement in PASI scores. The measures of quality of life also showed improvement. It is an important addition to the drugs that we have in treating psoriasis and psoriatic arthritis. However, treatment with leflunomide is not without side effects. Liver function tests have to be carried out and blood counts monitored monthly while on treatment. Blood pressure may increase. Severe diarrhoea may occur as well as skin rash. It is contraindicated in women with child-bearing potential due to high risk of teratogenicity.

Other DMARDs

Although not shown to protect from progression of joint damage, gold (both oral and by injection) has been used, with intramuscular gold being more effective. With significant concern about toxicity, slow mode of action, problems with availability, and availability of more effective drugs, it is seldom used nowadays. Penicillamine use is limited due to its toxicity. There are some reports that mycophenolate mofetil may be efficacious, but there have been no controlled clinical trials to prove its role. Etretinate (a retinoic acid derivative) has been shown to be effective in one controlled trial and two small uncontrolled trials.

DMARDs have traditionally been used as initial therapy in patients with peripheral psoriatic arthritis. However, a recent review of all available data concluded that there is lack of evidence that they are effective. There is some evidence that methotrexate, sulfasalazine, leflunomide, and cyclosporin A provide some symptom relief, but there is no evidence that they prevent disease progression and radiographic damage.

Myth

Treatment with DMARDs prevents joint damage.

 Fact

DMARDs have not been shown to prevent joint damage, although methotrexate, sulfasalazine, and cyclosporin A may improve symptoms.

Biological agents

Biological agents, especially anti-tumour necrosis factor (TNF) agents, have revolutionized the treatment of psoriatic arthritis. They have been shown to relieve symptoms and signs, and prevent further joint damage.

Anti-TNF agents

Infliximab

TNF is an important biological molecule that drives inflammation. Infliximab is a part human–part mouse antibody that binds to human TNF, and inactivates it. It is administered as an intravenous infusion at 0, 2, and 6 weeks, followed by once every 8 weeks. In controlled trials, infliximab was found to be remarkably effective in psoriatic arthritis. The Infliximab Multinational Psoriatic Arthritis Controlled Trial (IMPACT) has demonstrated that 65% of patients showed a significant improvement within 16 weeks of commencing treatment compared with only 10% of placebo-treated patients. Among patients who had PASI scores of 2.5 or more at baseline, 68% of infliximab-treated patients achieved improvement of 75% or more in the PASI score at week 16 compared with none of the placebo-treated patients. Sustained improvement was seen through week 50. Dactylitis and enthesitis also improved. Adverse events were similar between the treatment groups. The improvement persisted through 1 and 2 years of follow-up. The larger IMPACT 2 trial showed similar results to the IMPACT trial, with significant improvement in active psoriatic arthritis, psoriasis, dactylitis, and enthesitis. Both IMPACT and IMPACT 2 demonstrated a favourable effect of infliximab on progression of joint damage. Infliximab was shown to improve quality of life and function in patients with psoriatic arthritis.

Etanercept

Etanercept is a protein that binds to and inactivates TNF. It is administered as a subcutaneous injection twice weekly, the usual dose being 25 mg per dose. Etanercept was the first anti-TNF agent to be used in psoriatic arthritis. Results from the first phase II controlled trial in psoriatic arthritis showed that at 12 weeks 87% of etanercept-treated patients responded compared with 23% of placebo-treated patients. Injection site reactions were more common among the etanercept-treated patients. The results were further confirmed in a phase III multicentre trial, which also demonstrated significant sustained improvement in quality of life. There was also less radiographic progression. As in the previous trial, the only significant difference in the safety profile between etanercept and placebo was that there were more injection site reactions with etanercept. While the controlled clinical trials suggest that etanercept exerts its effect early, a recent observational study cautions that in some patients response may be delayed and noted only after 6 months of therapy. Etanercept has also shown a potential to prevent progression of joint damage, as well as to improve quality of life and function.

Adalimumab

Adalimumab is a fully human anti-TNF antibody and is administered subcutaneously at 2-weekly intervals. Results from the ADEPT trial, a phase III controlled clinical trial, showed that 57% of adalimumab-treated patients show a significant response at 24 weeks compared with 14% of placebo-treated patients. In those with more than 3% body surface area involvement with psoriasis, PASI 50/75/90 response was achieved in 75/59/42% of patients, respectively, compared with 12/1/0% in the placebo-treated patients. Adalimumab has also been reported to lead to clinically meaningful and statistically significant improvement in quality of life and function, as well as improvement in fatigue. It has also been shown to be effective in inhibiting radiographic disease progression. There was no difference in the adverse events between drug-treated and placebo-treated patient groups.

Adverse events

Adverse events due to treatment with anti-TNF agents can be significant. The most common side effects are injection site reactions to etanercept and adalimumab, and infusion reactions with infliximab. Injection site reactions are a nuisance, but infusion reactions may be life-threatening. The major side effect is increased risk of infection. Patients with active infections should not be treated with these agents. There is also a high risk of reactivation of latent tuberculosis or chronic fungal infections. Therefore, patients are screened for the presence of infections, especially tuberculosis, with a chest X-ray and the

TB skin test. If the chest X-ray shows evidence of past tuberculosis or if the skin test is positive, the risk of reactivation of tuberculosis needs to be assessed, ideally by an infectious disease specialist. If the risk is significant, a short course of treatment with anti-tuberculosis medications may be required. Treatment with anti-TNF agents may be commenced after the course of anti-tuberculosis medications is over or, if psoriatic arthritis is very active, after 1 month of treatment with anti-tuberculosis medications. Anti-TNF agents also worsen multiple sclerosis and should not be used in patients with this condition. Some patients have developed **demyelination** of the spinal cord, although the incidence is extremely rare. No increase in malignancy risk has been reported in patients with psoriatic arthritis. Another, curious side effect in patients treated with anti-TNF agents is the development of psoriasis, usually palmo-plantar pustulosis. This has also been noted in patients treated with anti-TNF agents for other diseases such as rheumatoid arthritis.

T cell-directed agents

Interactions such as those between lymphocyte function-associated antigen 1 (LFA-1) and its ligand intercellular adhesion molecule 1 (ICAM-1), and LFA-3 and CD2 are required for full T cell activation. Activated T cells are important in driving psoriasis and psoriatic arthritis. Molecules inhibiting these interactions have been developed recently.

Alefacept

Alefacept is a fully human fusion protein consisting of the first extracellular domain of LFA-3 fused to the hinge segment and constant regions of human IgG1. It inhibits antigen-driven activation of T cells and of memory T cells. A controlled trial of alefacept (15 mg once weekly by intramuscular injection) in combination with methotrexate in patients with active psoriatic arthritis despite treatment with methotrexate showed that at 24 weeks there was a significant response in 54% of alefacept-treated patients compared with 23% of patients on placebo. In patients with psoriasis involving more than 3% of the body surface area, 53% of alefacept-treated patients achieved PASI 50 compared with 17% of those receiving placebo. These results were obtained at 24 weeks, although the active drug was given for only the first 12 weeks of the study. Adverse events were mild to moderate and fewer than 2% of alefacept-treated patients discontinued treatment due to treatment-related adverse events. Side effects are chiefly due to infections. Treatment with alefacept leads to a steady decline in a subclass of T cells, called CD4 cells, that are important in the immune response. Therefore, CD4 counts have to be monitored weekly when on treatment with this drug, and the injections stopped if the levels fall below 250 cells/μl.

Efalizumab

Efalizumab is a humanized monoclonal IgG1 antibody against CD11a, one of the subunits of LFA-1. It is effective in the treatment of psoriasis. Results of a phase II trial with this agent for psoriatic arthritis have been disappointing, with only 28% of the patients achieving a significant response compared with 19% of the placebo-treated patients. Moreover, patients with psoriasis without psoriatic arthritis treated with efalizumab have developed new-onset inflammatory arthritis, and psoriatic arthritis has worsened in patients with psoriasis and psoriatic arthritis. Therefore, dermatologists do not prefer using this agent in patients with psoriatic arthritis.

Management of psoriatic arthritis today

With the availability of a large number of agents, with good efficacy and low toxicity, we have a number of options for treating patients with psoriatic arthritis. However, due to concerns about costs and long-term toxicity, the newer agents are being used cautiously.

Our approach to treatment of patients with psoriatic arthritis is based on a step-up strategy. Patients with mild psoriasis and arthritis are treated with topical agents and NSAIDs with or without intra-articular corticosteroids. Patients with evidence of persistent synovitis despite these measures, or those who have evidence of severe joint disease (three swollen joints, erosive disease), are first given an adequate trial with at least two DMARDs (methotrexate, leflunomide, sulfasalazine, or cyclosporin A). We define an adequate trial of methotrexate as the maximum tolerated dose, given either orally or parenterally (intramuscular or subcutaneous for doses >17.5 mg/week), for at least 3 months. Leflunomide is given at a dose of 20 mg daily. We prefer not to give the loading dose. Sulfasalazine up to 4 g/day for 3 months may be tried in patients who are not sensitive to the drug. Cyclosporin is given at a dose of 3–5 mg/kg with close monitoring of kidney and liver functions and blood pressure. If patients continue to have active joint disease (three or more tender and three or more swollen joints), an anti-TNF agent, usually etanercept or adalimumab, is instituted. If there is a failure on etanercept, infliximab or adalimumab is tried. Other biologicals are considered if the patient still does not respond.

If the patient's predominant symptoms are due to spondylitis (back disease) or enthesitis, treatment with traditional DMARDs is ineffective. In this situation we recommend that the patients be treated with a full therapeutic dose of NSAIDs. At least two different NSAIDs for 2 weeks have to be tried. If the patient continues to have significant symptoms after a trial with two different NSAIDs, he/she may be treated with anti-TNF agents, either etanercept, infliximab, or adalimumab (Fig. 10.1).

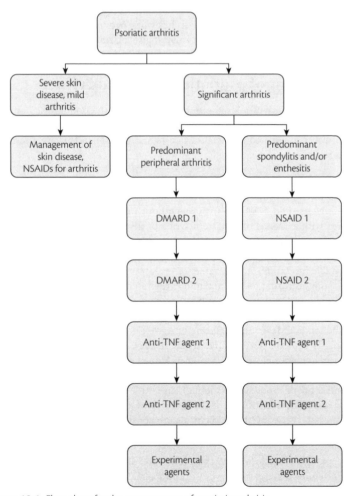

Figure 10.1 Flow chart for the management of psoriatic arthritis.

Summary

Psoriatic arthritis has the potential to cause destructive arthritis and has a significant impact on the functional capacity and health-related quality of life. Drugs with proven efficacy are available for its management today. Biological agents have better efficacy than the traditional DMARDs, and prevent progression of joint damage. Further clinical studies are required, however, to define clearly their place in management of patients with psoriatic arthritis given their cost and concerns for long-term safety.

11

Surgery in psoriatic arthritis

 Key points

- Joint deformities and damage occur in a substantial number of patients with psoriatic arthritis

- These deformities are related to the degree of joint inflammation

- Ideally patients should be treated early to control inflammation and thus prevent progression of joint damage

- Several surgical procedures are available for patients with psoriatic arthritis

Deformities and damage in psoriatic arthritis

Psoriatic arthritis is an inflammatory arthritis associated with psoriasis. The arthritis presents with tender and swollen joints, and in about half the patients there is involvement of the spine, with pain, stiffness, and limitation of movement. The inflammation in the affected area may lead to deformities and damage if it is not controlled. Although many patients complain of joint pain and seek medical attention, as a group patients with psoriatic arthritis do not complain of as much pain as patients with other forms of arthritis. For that reason, many patients only realize that they have a problem once they have developed joint deformities. It was found that 67% of the patients presenting to psoriatic arthritis clinics after 9 years of disease have at least one joint showing erosions on X-rays. Another study showed that some 20% of the patients present to a clinic with five or more deformed joints, again after a disease duration of approximately 9 years. After 10 years of follow-up, 55% of the patients have five or more deformed joints. Thus, the disease has a propensity to lead to joint damage. Studies have revealed that persistent joint inflammation is associated with both clinical and radiological damage.

Types of joint damage in psoriatic arthritis

There are several types of joint damage which can occur in patients with psoriatic arthritis. Joint damage may be detected clinically, when the physician examines the patients. On the other hand, joint damage may not be apparent clinically, but may be detected radiologically, when X-rays are taken. While there is a correlation between clinical and radiological damage when severe X-ray changes occur, clinical deformities may not be apparent when only erosions are present without any evidence of joint space narrowing.

Joint deformities

A deformity is noted when the joint demonstrates marked reduction in the range of movement. Joints may develop **contractures** where they are stuck in one position, usually bent, and are not able to straighten out (Fig. 11.1). This commonly occurs in the small joints of the hands and feet, but may also affect large joints such as the wrists, elbows, knees, and hips. This deformity often results from scarring of the joints. Later on, bony bridging across the joint

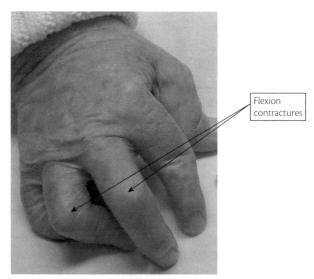

Flexion contractures

Figure 11.1 Flexion contractures limiting hand function in psoriatic arthritis.

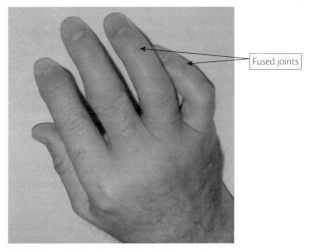

Figure 11.2 Ankylosed joints in psoriatic arthritis.

may occur, and the joint becomes fused, or totally ankylosed (Fig. 11.2). Another common deformity in patients with psoriatic arthritis is **flail joints** (Fig. 11.3, p. 92). This usually results from total destruction of the joint and leads to instability of the joint. This may occur in any of the joints of the hands and feet. Joint deformities may lead to impaired function and disability depending on what position the joint is in once it has developed the deformity. Another deformity which occurs primarily in the hands and feet joints is **subluxation**, where one bone falls off the other, making the joint totally dysfunctional (Fig. 11.4, p. 93). Thus, some joints with deformity may still allow function, albeit reduced, while other deformed joints lead to dysfunction.

Predictors of joint damage in psoriatic arthritis

Studies have shown that the factors that predict joint damage are the degree of joint inflammation, as measured by the number of tender and swollen joints, as well as the presence of blood markers of inflammation such as an elevated erythrocyte sedimentation rate (ESR) or C-reactive protein (CRP). Thus, ideally patients should be treated for the acute inflammation early, to avoid development of joint destruction. Once such joint damage has occurred, the benefit from medical therapy is limited, and surgical approaches may be more appropriate.

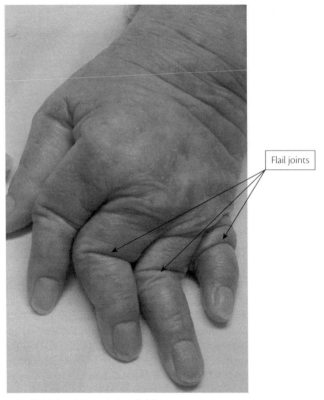

Flail joints

Figure 11.3 Flail joints in psoriatic arthritis.

Indications for surgery in psoriatic arthritis

The indications for surgery in patients with psoriatic arthritis are similar to those of patients with other forms of arthritis. One main indication is persistent pain, which is thought to arise from mechanical rather than inflammatory mechanisms. The other is functional limitation. Surgery is therefore performed when patients have severe pain in a joint which has been deformed or where there has been marked cartilage destruction. These joints will probably not respond to medical therapies, and therefore the only approach would be to operate.

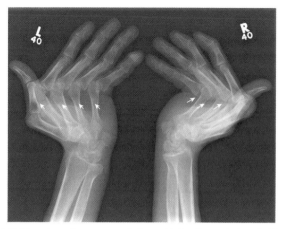

Figure 11.4 Subluxation of metacarpophalangeal joints in psoriatic arthritis.

Surgical procedures

Several surgical procedures may be required for patients with psoriatic arthritis. Those may involve the peripheral joints of the hands and feet, larger joints such as knees, hips, and shoulders, and in some cases the spine. Most operations are performed for pain relief, particularly in the hips and knees, as well as the back. Some surgeries are performed for disability resulting from the deformities and joint damage. On occasion when a particular joint demonstrates persistent inflammation, and medical therapy, including joint injections, has not helped, a surgical **synovectomy** is performed. This type of surgery removes the lining of the joint (**synovium**) which theoretically should remove the inflamed area within the particular joint. Synovectomies were commonly performed years ago, when the medical treatment of arthritis was not that effective. However, with the advent of better medical therapies, it has not been performed commonly in recent years.

Surgery for the small joints of the hands and feet

As noted above, there are three major deformities in the small joints of the hands and feet in psoriatic arthritis. These include flexion **contractures** or bending of the joints. This may occur in the end joints (distal) of the hands and feet, in which case patients may manage with activities of daily living despite the deformity, and surgery may not be required. However, if such changes occur in the middle joints of the fingers (proximal interphalangeal joints), or in the joints between the fingers and the hand (metacarpophalangeal joints), they interfere with function, and surgery may be indicated. At times, procedures which straighten the bones or osteotomies have been performed with varying results. There are no specific studies of these procedures in patients with psoriatic arthritis. These procedures are not usually performed on the small joints of the hands or feet. Often the surgeon will break the bones and fuse them in a more functional position.

Another deformity, loosening of the joints or 'flail joints', may lead to dysfunction particularly in the hands since they may result in a patient's inability to grasp things. In such cases the operation of choice is fusion of the affected joint to make it immobile and thus more stable and functional.

Another type of surgery that may be performed is joint replacement. However, joint replacements in the small joints of the hands have not been particularly successful in patients with psoriatic arthritis since there tends to be a bony reaction which leads to flexion contractures and fusion. Similar attempts to correct the original flexion contractures or **joint fusion** with joint replacement in the small joints of the hands have also led to subsequent bony proliferation around the prosthesis and resulted in the same problem of joint contracture and limited mobility.

As noted, joint subluxation occurs when the bones around the joint lose their usual contact and one bone positions itself either above or below the other, or on one side or the other. The result of subluxation is that the affected fingers or toes are twisted to one side or the other. This type of deformity clearly results in functional impairment. Most of the time joint replacement surgery is performed for this deformity and may provide better contact between the bones around the joint. Again, there is concern regarding risk of failure of this surgery because of the bony proliferation.

Surgery for knee and hip joints

Knee and hip surgery is often done for pain, usually the result of cartilage loss and bone rubbing on bone. In this instance, two possible procedures may be performed. If the cartilage is lost on only one of the bones which make up the joint, the surgeon may decide to cover that area with a 'spacer' and not do anything to the other bone if it appears normal. These procedures are called hemiarthroplasty, since they only apply to half of the joint. In the hip, sometimes the surgeon only replaces the femur, or hip bone, and does not do anything to the acetabulum, which is the socket where the femur articulates. Occasionally the acetabulum is lined when the femur does not need replacement.

In the knee, at times only the femur may be covered, with the tibia being left intact. At other times the femur is left intact and the tibial plateau is resurfaced.

As total joint replacement surgery has improved over the years, in terms of both the prostheses developed and advances in the surgical procedure itself, more and more joint replacements are being done. Nowadays, the majority of procedures performed on knees and hips are total joint replacements. Total joint replacement surgery in psoriatic arthritis is usually successful, and in many patients the prostheses last more than a decade. Synovectomies are still performed on occasion when there is thickened synovium which does not respond to medical therapy.

Experience with surgical procedures in psoriatic arthritis

There are few studies addressing surgery in patients with psoriatic arthritis. In a pathology study it was reported many years ago that the joints of patients with psoriatic arthritis were scarred. A report in 1952 showed that surgery on these joints could help by reducing the scar tissue. One study demonstrated that about 7% of the patients followed over time required surgery and that the likelihood of surgery increased with disease duration. In that study, the average disease duration at the time of surgery was 13 years. The most common surgical procedure was total hip replacement, followed by total knee replacement. Joint replacement in the metacarpophalangeal joints (the knuckles closest to the hand) was also performed, followed by fusion surgery for the fingers, wrists, and ankles. A few patients had synovectomies, including knee, wrist, and elbow. One patient had realignment of the metacarpophalangeal joint without having joint replacement. The majority of the patients had only one procedure, but in 28% several procedures were performed. The upper and lower extremities were involved in a similar number of patients, with few patients having both upper and lower extremity surgery. Surgery was predicted by the number of actively inflamed joints and the extent of damage seen on X-ray at presentation to the clinic. Patients with the highest number of severely affected joints both clinically and on X-rays were more likely to have surgery. Although patients who had surgery had more severe disease, their health outcomes were not worse than non-surgery patients, suggesting that the surgery was done for legitimate indications and at least helped the patients to maintain a reasonable level of health and function.

In another study, the type and outcome of reconstructive surgery for different patterns of psoriatic arthritis over a 10-year period was studied. The patients were divided into three groups: distal joint involvement, oligoarticular (less than five joints), and polyarticular (five or more joints involved). It was shown that the majority of patients had polyarticular disease. The majority of the operations done in this group of patients included complex hand and foot reconstruction, followed by hip replacements, and surgical fusion of different joints. In the oligoarticular group, most of the procedures involved joint replacement, usually the hip or knee. Patients with distal arthritis had fusions in the distal joints. Patients with polyarticular disease had a lower level of physical functioning according to the scores on the physical function domain of a quality of life questionnaire.

Spinal surgery

In addition to the peripheral arthritis, patients with psoriatic arthritis also have involvement of the joints of the spine. Patients with severe psoriatic spondylitis may develop marked deformity of the spine and on occasion require surgery to correct this deformity. While there are no reported studies specifically describing spinal surgery in patients with psoriatic arthritis, the procedures are similar to those performed in patients with ankylosing spondylitis.

Surgery other than joint surgery in psoriatic arthritis

Patients with psoriatic arthritis also undergo a variety of surgical procedures which individuals without psoriatic arthritis may require. The difficulty for patients with psoriatic arthritis is that they have psoriasis, which may cause complications. First, the surgeon must avoid cutting through a psoriatic plaque so that infection does not set in. In addition, psoriasis may interfere with skin healing, and patients with psoriatic arthritis may be on immunosuppressive medications which may also hinder healing. Even NSAIDs may have an effect on bleeding as well as wound healing. For that reason, it is important for patients with psoriatic arthritis to consult their rheumatologist before undergoing any type of surgery, so that appropriate drug management may be carried out. Drugs such as methotrexate and the new biological agents are usually held over the operative period. Anti-inflammatory medications such as aspirin and related compounds are held for 7–10 days to avoid excessive bleeding.

12

A team approach

Relationship between skin and joint disease in psoriatic arthritis

Psoriasis is a chronic inflammatory skin disease which affects 2–3% of the population. Among patients suffering from psoriasis, about 30% will develop an inflammatory form of arthritis called psoriatic arthritis. Many investigators believe that patients with severe psoriasis are more likely to develop arthritis than patients with mild disease. However, it is still not clear that this is the case. Patients seen in rheumatology clinics usually do not have severe psoriasis, and some patients do not have psoriasis at all and yet present with psoriatic arthritis. Moreover, there is no direct relationship between the extent of psoriasis and the severity of the arthritis. Thus, patients may have mild psoriasis and mild arthritis, mild psoriasis and severe arthritis, severe psoriasis and mild arthritis, and severe psoriasis and severe arthritis. It is important for patients with psoriasis who develop arthritis to be diagnosed early, and obtain appropriate medical care, since the extent and severity of arthritis at presentation have been shown to predict progression of joint deformities and radiological damage, as well as early mortality. In order to arrive at the correct diagnosis early, a team approach to the management of psoriatic arthritis must prevail.

The team approach

The team consists of the patient, the primary care physician, the dermatologist, and the rheumatologist, as well as allied health professionals including nurses, physiotherapists, occupational therapists, and pharmacists. It is unusual for patients to present to a specialist without a referral from a primary care physician, usually a general practitioner or family physician.

How does the primary care or family physician help a patient with psoriasis?

The family physician is the point of entry into the health care system. Patients should therefore report to the primary care or family physician if they have a skin rash or joint complaints. While psoriasis is quite variable and many primary care physicians can easily treat mild psoriasis with topical medications, patients who have moderate to severe psoriasis should be referred to a dermatologist. Patients who have psoriasis in areas difficult to treat such as the scalp, the face, the anal cleft, or the groin would benefit from seeing a dermatologist. Patients with psoriasis who report to the primary care physician and the dermatologist may be referred to a rheumatologist if they have any joint pain or swelling, any limitation of joint movement, or any back pain or stiffness. These complaints may indicate that psoriatic arthritis is developing. Once the primary care physician is aware of these complaints, they may seek advice from a rheumatologist who will make the correct diagnosis and provide a management plan.

Can psoriatic arthritis be detected in the absence of psoriasis?

About 15% of patients who ultimately are diagnosed with psoriatic arthritis present with their joint manifestations before their skin disease. A diagnosis of psoriatic arthritis may be more difficult in this situation. However, the diagnosis can still be made if the patient presents with typical features of psoriatic arthritis even if they do not have psoriasis. These features include the involvement of the end joints (distal joints) of the fingers or toes, the presence of inflammation at the insertion of tendons into bones (enthesitis), or the presence of a swollen finger or toe (dactylitis). A rheumatologist may be able to make the diagnosis of psoriatic arthritis even in the absence of psoriasis. It is therefore important that patients with joint complaints relate these complaints to their primary physician who may then refer them to a rheumatologist to arrive at the correct diagnosis of their joint manifestations. It is also important for patients to tell their physicians if they have any family members with psoriasis, since that facilitates the diagnosis.

When should a patient see a dermatologist?

When the patient presents with joint manifestations without skin disease, it is important to report whether there are family members affected with psoriasis. The rheumatologist, once presented with the unique manifestations of psoriatic arthritis, will probably pay specific attention to skin and nail changes and may refer patients to a dermatologist to confirm the diagnosis of these lesions. Once a diagnosis is confirmed, the follow-up of a patient should probably include both dermatologist and rheumatologist. These physicians may decide who should be following the patient more closely. Generally this will depend on the most significant problem for the patient. If the psoriasis is severe, or occurs in areas that are hard to treat, the dermatologist may be the primary specialist to follow the patient, seeking advice for the joint disease management as necessary. However, if the joint manifestations are the main issue, the rheumatologist will probably be the primary specialist, and the dermatologist be consulted as necessary.

Role of other health professionals

The nurse may be required to administer medications for both the skin and joints. The physiotherapist and occupational therapist may be required to address an exercise programme and maintenance of functional ability, as well as provide splints where indicated. The pharmacist will ultimately provide the medications for the patients. It is most important that the patient understands the effect of medications including therapeutic effects and side effects, medication interactions, and the effect of unrelated medications on the skin.

Is the team available everywhere?

While the above seems like a rational and simple approach, this system is not in operation in many parts of the world. Indeed, even in the developed world, the team approach has not been instituted. In many countries there are shortages of dermatologists and rheumatologists. The shortage in specialists in this area may result from the fact that medical students may not be exposed to rheumatologists and dermatologists early in the course of their studies, and may have already determined their future career by the time that exposure occurs. In developed countries, physicians opt for more glamorous specialties such as cardiology, nephrology, and gastroenterology. Even if physicians choose dermatology as their specialty, they prefer to perform cosmetic dermatology rather than medical dermatology. In developing countries, other conditions are much more urgent than psoriasis and arthritis. They are still trying to control infectious diseases and therefore these conditions take a second or third place in the medical care. Even if there are sufficient numbers of physicians in both specialties, there are many areas where dermatologists and rheumatologists do not work together. Thus it is difficult to establish the team to look after the patients.

Moreover, some physicians do not perceive psoriasis as a health issue. It is common, and it is 'only a rash'. It is not perceived as a life-threatening condition, although it has become clear from studies in the past 10–15 years that psoriasis has a major effect on quality of life. While patients with severe psoriasis may be referred early to a dermatologist, those with milder forms may not be. Although some have suggested that patients with more severe psoriasis may develop psoriatic arthritis, it is clear from the studies performed in psoriatic arthritis clinics that the majority of patients with psoriatic arthritis do not have severe psoriasis. Thus it may be that the patients with milder psoriasis need to be investigated for the presence of arthritis. There are several groups working on the development of screening questionnaires and instruments which will help dermatologists and primary care physicians to identify patients with psoriasis who are destined to develop arthritis.

How are health professionals trained in the team approach?

It should be noted that the training in each of the specialties relevant to the assessment of patients with psoriatic arthritis is different. Dermatologists are trained in the diagnosis and management of skin disease. They are not trained to assess actively inflamed or damaged joints. Rheumatologists on the other hand are trained in assessing and managing joint disease and are not trained to diagnose or treat skin disease. Physicians select their respective specialty because of interest in the particular topic, and it would be inappropriate to expect that they should be including each other's assessment tools in the day to day management of their patients. Nonetheless, in some randomized clinical trials, dermatologists have been expected to perform the assessment of joint disease while rheumatologists have been carrying out skin assessments.

The International Multicentre Psoriasis and Arthritis Reproducibility Trial (IMPART)

A recent study performed under the auspices of the Group for Research and Assessment of Psoriasis and Psoriatic Arthritis (GRAPPA) tested the degree of agreement among rheumatologists and dermatologists in assessing skin and joint manifestations in psoriatic arthritis. The study included ten rheumatologists and ten dermatologists who assessed 20 patients with psoriatic arthritis who had different degrees of skin and joint manifestations. Each patient was seen by the same ten observers, half of whom were dermatologists and half of whom were rheumatologists. The study showed that there was very good agreement in the assessment of tender joints, but not swollen joints. While there was a good agreement among rheumatologists on the assessment of dactylitis (sausage digits), there was very poor agreement among dermatologists on that aspect. There was excellent agreement among rheumatologists and dermatologists on the assessment of nail involvement, both in terms of the number of nails involved and in terms of a specific instrument to score the degree of nail involvement. Dermatologists and rheumatologists had very good agreement on the psoriasis area and severity index (PASI), a measure commonly used to assess psoriasis. Dermatologists had better agreement about other measures to assess skin disease, although rheumatologists also had pretty good agreement. The physician global assessment was not a good instrument for rheumatologists, whether it was for joints or skin. While dermatologists demonstrated better agreement than rheumatologists, it was not as good as for the specific instruments. It was concluded from the study that further training was required in order to achieve better agreement, and that an education programme needs to be developed to teach medical students and physicians in training how to assess skin and joint disease in psoriatic arthritis.

GRAPPA provides an opportunity for rheumatologists and dermatologists to work together to develop teams in various sites. Once the two specialists work together, they can incorporate the other health care professionals into the team.

Other issues needing to be addressed

It may indeed be necessary for other health care professionals to join the team of professionals looking after patients with psoriatic arthritis. This is because there are other medical problems that seem to affect patients with psoriatic arthritis more than the general population. Patients with psoriatic arthritis are more prone to obesity, high blood pressure, and have a higher prevalence of heart attacks than the general population. Therefore, endocrinologists and cardiologists may be necessary to address these issues.

13

Lessons from the University of Toronto Psoriatic Arthritis Clinic

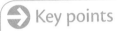 Key points

- A well characterized **longitudinal observational cohort** provides important information on the course and prognosis of psoriatic arthritis

- Disease progression in psoriatic arthritis is related to previous disease activity and damage

- There is an increased risk of death among patients with psoriatic arthritis which is related to previous disease activity and damage

- There are patients with psoriatic arthritis who go into prolonged remission

- There are several genetic factors predisposing to psoriatic arthritis

The development of the Psoriatic Arthritis Clinic

The University of Toronto Psoriatic Arthritis Clinic has provided a unique opportunity to study the course and prognosis of psoriatic arthritis as well as its pathogenesis and management. The Clinic was established by Dr Dafna Gladman in 1978, when it became apparent to her that the understanding of this disease was minimal. In 1976, an elaborate outpatient facility for patients with psoriasis was established by the late Dr Ricky Kanee Schachter at Women's College Hospital in Toronto, Canada. The Psoriasis Education and Research Centre (PERC) was established as an outpatient centre for the assessment, education, and treatment of patients with psoriasis. As a newly appointed rheumatologist at Women's College Hospital, Dr Gladman was asked to consult at PERC as the staff noted that many of the patients suffered not only from psoriasis, but also from its associated arthritis. Dr Gladman noticed that patients suffering from psoriatic arthritis had a very severe form of arthritis which progressed rapidly. This was contrary to the teaching she had received during her training. She therefore embarked on a study to determine the course and prognosis of psoriatic arthritis and established the University of Toronto Psoriatic Arthritis Clinic.

Assessment of psoriatic arthritis patients at the Psoriatic Arthritis Clinic

Patients with an inflammatory arthritis associated with psoriasis have been entered into the Clinic since 1 January 1978, and their longitudinal information has been tracked electronically and made available for statistical analyses.

A standard protocol has been developed to allow collection of similar information from all patients. The protocol includes details of the development of the disease in each patient, including age of onset of skin and joint manifestations, family history of psoriasis, psoriatic arthritis, and other related forms of arthritis. Other demographic features recorded included the ethnic background, whether patients had had an infection or trauma prior to the onset of their skin and joint disease, and whether they had smoked or consumed alcohol. The marital status and employment status were also recorded at the time of the onset of the disease. The presence of infection and trauma in the interim period is recorded at each visit, as is the marital status, employment status, smoking, and alcohol consumption. A complete medical history is obtained at each visit, which includes information on other co-morbid conditions such as cardiovascular disease, diabetes, and cancer. A detailed history of peripheral arthritis and spinal disease is included. History of the joint pain and swelling, morning stiffness, neck and back pain and stiffness, evidence of sausage digits (dactylitis), and pain at the insertion of tendons into bone (enthesitis) is collected at each visit. A very detailed drug history is obtained. Treatment of both skin and joint disease is recorded, as well as treatment for other conditions. A complete physical examination is recorded, as well as skin and joint manifestations, and back and neck mobility. All these measurements are done in a standard way which has been proven reliable in the Clinic. Additionally, patients undergo routine laboratory evaluations at each Clinic visit, and radiographic evaluation at 2-year intervals. Patients also complete questionnaires pertaining to their quality of life and function, and the effect of both skin and joint manifestations on their daily life.

Upon entering the Clinic, patients give consent allowing the information collected to be used in analyses, and also consent to provide additional blood samples for specialized laboratory tests including genetic analyses. All the information collected on the patients with psoriatic arthritis is entered onto an ORACLE database. Thus, longitudinal information is available for statistical analyses evaluating the disease course, use of therapies, and outcomes in these patients.

Validation of the measures assessed in the Clinic

Several physicians assess the patients at the University of Toronto Psoriatic Arthritis Clinic. Each year there are Rheumatology Specialty Residents from the University of Toronto Rheumatology Training Program assigned to the Clinic for a 6–12 month period. In addition there are clinical research fellows who attend the Clinic for 1–2 years at a time. These research trainees come from all over the world to obtain further training both in psoriatic arthritis and in database research. In addition, many students, both undergraduates and graduates, have participated in the studies performed at the University of Toronto Psoriatic Arthritis Clinic. Several of these students obtained their degrees through the studies they carried out in the Clinic.

In order to ensure that the clinical measures used to assess the patients in the Clinic were performed in a similar manner by the physicians working in the Clinic, we conducted a reliability study. Several individuals who had worked in the Clinic as well as Dr Gladman assessed the same patients in a specific format. The design allowed the assessment of the contribution of the patient differences, the order of the examination, and the differences among assessors to the variability of the results. The results of the analysis confirmed that the assessment of actively inflamed and clinically damaged joints by these physicians was almost identical. Subsequently a study comparing the radiological scoring system used in the Clinic by a rheumatologist and a radiologist confirmed their agreement, as well as their ability to determine changes over time. Thus we could use the information collected prospectively in our studies on prognosis.

Effect of loss to follow-up

It was initially thought that patients attending a special clinic for psoriatic arthritis would be worse than patients seen in other clinics. Moreover, it was thought that patients referred to the Clinic early would be much worse as physicians might have referred to the Clinic those patients that they had most difficulty with. Patients who were referred in the first 5 years of the Clinic were therefore compared with the patients referred in the second 5 years. No differences were detected in the clinical, laboratory, or radiological features among these patients. It was important to make sure that patients who continued to be followed at the Clinic were not different from those who elected not to continue follow-up at the Clinic. The clinical, laboratory, and radiographic features of patients who were followed in the Clinic regularly were compared with those of patients who were lost to follow-up to ensure that there was no selection of patients with more severe disease to remain in the Clinic. No differences were identified, suggesting that there was no bias towards patients with more severe disease in the longitudinal cohort. In addition, patients who had not attended the Clinic for more than 2 years were recalled, and their clinical, laboratory, and radiological features were compared with those of patients who were followed regularly. There were no differences among patients followed regularly and those who were lost to follow-up either at first or at last visit; there was also no difference among patients who returned to Clinic and those who were unable to attend. Thus, there did not appear to be a systematic problem with the patients who were being followed at the Clinic. We were now ready to examine questions related to the course and prognosis of this disease.

Disease severity

The first study published from the psoriatic arthritis longitudinal cohort confirmed the original observation by Dr Gladman and the reason for establishing the Clinic. It demonstrated that psoriatic arthritis was indeed more severe than previously thought. This study was published in 1987 and was based on the first 220 patients registered in the Psoriatic Arthritis Clinic. There were 116 females and 104 males, a ratio of 1.1 to 1, which is similar to other reported series. The mean age at the first visit to the Clinic was 46 years. The average age of onset of psoriasis was 29 years, while that of psoriatic arthritis was 37 years. The average disease duration of psoriatic arthritis at first clinic visit was 9 years. The majority (68%) developed their psoriatic arthritis an average of 12.8 years after the onset of psoriasis; 15% presented with skin and joint manifestations at the same time, while in 17% the arthritis came before the psoriasis by an average of 7.4 years. Of the 220 patients, 67% already had evidence of radiological damage at their first visit to the Clinic. The study showed that 20% of these patients had a severe deforming arthritis and 11% had significant functional disability. Most of the patients had polyarticular disease (involving five or more joints) and 34% had back involvement. Only 2% of the patients had back disease without any peripheral joint disease. Patients with back involvement were older at the time of onset of their arthritis than patients without back involvement.

Assessment of tenderness in patients with psoriatic arthritis

Patients with psoriatic arthritis were compared with those with rheumatoid arthritis in terms of pain perception. The study documented that patients with psoriatic arthritis did not experience as much tenderness as patients with rheumatoid arthritis. The study compared the ability of patients with psoriatic arthritis and patients with rheumatoid arthritis to tolerate pain as measured by a special instrument called a dolorimeter. This instrument allows one to measure the degree of pressure that can be applied to a particular point before a person pulls away because of pain. The amount of pressure that could be applied to the most actively inflamed joint, a control point, and a fibromyalgia tender point was measured in kilograms.

Fibromyalgia tender points are points in the body which are very tender in individuals with the fibromyalgia syndrome. The fibromyalgia syndrome consists of extreme fatigue, pain all over, lack of deep sleep, as well as other features. Since this syndrome can affect patients with arthritis, it was relevant to measure fibromyalgia tender points in patients with psoriatic arthritis. It was found that fibromyalgia was less common in patients with psoriatic arthritis than in patients with rheumatoid arthritis. The study indicated that one could press almost twice as hard on an inflamed joint of a patient with psoriatic arthritis as on an inflamed joint of a patient with rheumatoid arthritis. Moreover, one could press twice as hard on fibromyalgia tender points as well as on control points in patients with psoriatic arthritis as on those with rheumatoid arthritis. This study thus documented that patients with psoriatic arthritis experienced less tenderness than patients with rheumatoid arthritis. This might explain why patients with psoriatic arthritis had been considered to have a mild disease, and why any of them did not present to a physician until they already had clinical damage.

Comparison between psoriatic arthritis and rheumatoid arthritis

Studies performed at the University of Toronto Psoriatic Arthritis Clinic demonstrated that the radiographic changes noted in psoriatic arthritis were as severe as those noted in rheumatoid arthritis patients. In addition, patients with psoriatic arthritis, like those with rheumatoid arthritis, had reduced quality of life and function.

Comparison between psoriatic arthritis and ankylosing spondylitis

As involvement of the spinal joints is a common feature of psoriatic arthritis, occurring in at least half of the patients, it was important to determine whether the spinal disease is different from that of ankylosing spondylitis. Ankylosing spondylitis is the prototype inflammatory disease of the back. It affects men more than women, usually in the late teens or early twenties. If untreated, it leads to marked spinal deformities and disability. Studies at the University of Toronto Psoriatic Arthritis Clinic documented that patients with psoriatic arthritis and spinal disease did not complain of as much pain and did not have the same degree of limitation of movement as patients with ankylosing spondylitis. Moreover, the radiological features were not as severe. This finding was recently confirmed by another study which compared the patients with psoriatic spondylitis followed in the Psoriatic Arthritis Clinic with those with ankylosing spondylitis followed at the spondylitis clinic at the Toronto Western Hospital.

Relationship of psoriatic arthritis to nail disease

A comparison between 158 patients with psoriatic arthritis and 101 patients with psoriasis who did not have arthritis was carried out in the University of Toronto Psoriatic Arthritis Clinic. The study demonstrated that the only clinical feature which distinguished the two groups was the presence of nail lesions, which occurred in 87% of the patients with psoriatic arthritis and only 46% of the patients with uncomplicated psoriasis. This has been confirmed by other studies and has been accepted by the International Psoriasis Council as a feature of psoriatic arthritis.

Change in arthritis pattern over time

The initial description of psoriatic arthritis included five clinical patterns: (1) distal joint disease (the involvement of the end joints of the fingers and toes); (2) oligoarthritis (involvement of four joints or less, usually in an asymmetric distribution); (3) polyarthritis (involvement of five or more joints, which may be symmetric and resemble rheumatoid arthritis); (4) primarily spinal involvement (where the joints of the spine were primarily involved); and (5) arthritis mutilans (a very destructive form of arthritis). However, when the University of Toronto Psoriatic Arthritis Clinic was established, it became clear that these arthritis patterns were not mutually exclusive. Thus, at the University of Toronto Psoriatic Arthritis Clinic the patterns were described as: distal, oligoarthritis, polyarthritis, back only, back with distal involvement, back with oligoarthritis, and back with polyarthritis. Arthritis mutilans was considered a description which could fit any of the other patterns. Moreover, it was noted that during follow-up patients may change from one pattern to another. Thus, patients may first present with distal joint disease but develop disease in other joints later on. They often do not have back disease at presentation, but develop it later on. Some patients may initially present with back disease but later develop peripheral joint disease. Indeed a study from the University of Toronto Psoriatic Arthritis Clinic showed that a change in arthritis pattern does occur over time. Also, it was noted that the arthritis pattern description was dependent on whether or not radiographs were performed. Many patients with psoriatic arthritis do not know that they have back involvement until X-rays are taken, since many of them do not complain of back pain. This study suggested that the definition of arthritis patterns to identify patients with psoriatic arthritis was only useful at presentation, and that perhaps the arthritis patterns should not be used in established disease.

Classification of psoriatic arthritis

The University of Toronto Psoriatic Arthritis Clinic was an important contributor to the international study of classification of psoriatic arthritis (CASPAR). This study included 30 investigators from 17 countries. The study led to the development of classification criteria for psoriatic arthritis which proved to be almost 99% specific and 91% sensitive for the classification of this disease. The criteria may be applied to individuals who have inflammatory arthritis, inflammatory spinal disease, or inflammation at the insertion of tendons into bone (enthesitis). Based on items listed in Table 13.1, if an individual accumulates 3 points they may be classified as having psoriatic arthritis. Using these criteria would facilitate including patients in drug trials and observational cohorts.

Further studies at the University of Toronto Psoriatic Arthritis Clinic confirmed that the CASPAR criteria are sensitive in patients with early psoriatic arthritis, and they are both sensitive and specific when applied in a family medicine clinic. Thus, the CASPAR criteria may be useful in the diagnosis of psoriatic arthritis.

Disease progression

Studies from the Psoriatic Arthritis Clinic demonstrated that over the follow-up period there was progression of both peripheral arthritis and back disease. Thus, in a study that included only patients who had evidence of back involvement, both peripheral joints and the spine showed progression over a 30-month period. Another study that looked at patients followed in the Clinic

Table 13.1 Classification criteria for psoriatic arthritis

Item	Score
Evidence of psoriasis	
Current psoriasis OR	2 OR
Past history OR	1 OR
Family history	1
Nail lesions	1
Dactylitis	
Current dactylitis OR	1 OR
History documented by rheumatologist	1
Negative rheumatoid factor	1
Evidence of fluffy periosteal reaction on X-ray	1
Total possible	6

for at least 5 years showed that the progression was faster early on, and that over time the rapidity of progression was reduced, suggesting that psoriatic arthritis tends to progress rapidly early in the course, and supporting the notion that patients should be diagnosed and treated early. Moreover, it was shown that by the time patients were followed for 10 years or more, 55% had developed at least five deformed joints. Studies from other centres subsequently supported these findings. Indeed, a study from an early arthritis clinic in Dublin showed that 47% of patients with psoriatic arthritis diagnosed within 5 months of onset of symptoms developed joint damage within 2 years of diagnosis, despite the fact that 56% of the patients had been treated with antirheumatic drugs. Thus by the mid-1990s it was clear that psoriatic arthritis was indeed a severe disease.

Predictors for progression of joint damage in psoriatic arthritis

Once it was shown that patients with psoriatic arthritis may have severe disease that progressed over time, it was necessary to identify the predictors of progression of damage. The initial study from the University of Toronto Psoriatic Arthritis Clinic to look at predictors for progression of joint damage looked specifically at clinical damage, which was assessed at each Clinic visit.

This study looked only at items present at the first Clinic visit as predictors. The study identified a high swollen joint count and a high medication level at presentation to Clinic as predictors of progression of clinical damage, while a low **erythrocyte sedimentation rate** (ESR), a measure of inflammation, was 'protective'. A further study added genetic markers to the clinical model. **HLA antigens** are molecules present on the cell surface, which are known to be associated with psoriasis and psoriatic arthritis. Those HLA antigens previously found to be associated with psoriasis and psoriatic arthritis were included in the first study. HLA-B27 in the presence of HLA-DR7, HLA-B39, and HLA-DQw3 in the absence of HLA-DR7 were found to be predictive of joint damage, and remained in the model even when the clinical features were added. An additional study which included all HLA antigens tested for identified HLA-B22 as protective from progression of clinical joint damage.

A further study which included not only features present at presentation to Clinic, but allowed features to vary with time, identified the number of actively inflamed joints at each visit, the number of damaged joints, and a high ESR as predictive of progression of clinical damage. Thus, it was clear that inflammation led to damage, and previous damage was also predictive of future damage. Subsequent studies determined that radiological damage preceded clinical damage.

In a subsequent study, the aim was to identify predictors for the development of radiological damage. It turned out that the same features predicted the progression of clinical and radiological damage: a high ESR, the number of tender and swollen joints, and the number of clinically damaged joints. Thus, for both clinical and radiological damage progression, disease activity and current damage are important, suggesting once again that earlier treatment would prevent progression of joint disease. What is very interesting with regards to these observations is the fact that in recent drug trials it has been shown that patients who had high levels of inflammation detected by the C-reactive protein were more susceptible to progression of joint damage detected radiologically within 6 months of the beginning of a drug trial. These observations support the findings from the longitudinal cohort.

Mortality in psoriatic arthritis

As patients were followed over time in the University of Toronto Psoriatic Arthritis Clinic, some deaths were identified. A question arose as to whether there was an increased risk for death among patients with psoriatic arthritis. The first study, which was published in 1997, reported that patients enrolled in the Clinic between 1978 and 1993 had an increased risk of death. Of the

428 patients with psoriatic arthritis enrolled by January 1993, 53 died by September 1994. The four leading causes of death were diseases of the circulatory (36.2%) or respiratory system (21.3%), malignant neoplasm (17.0%), and injuries/poisoning (14.9%). The overall standardized mortality ratio (SMR, a measure which compares the observed with the expected deaths in the group) was 1.62 (1.59 for females and 1.65 for men).

The predictors for death among the patients with psoriatic arthritis were severe disease at presentation and radiological damage, as well as a high ESR. These results highlight once again that active and severe disease leads to bad outcomes in patients with psoriatic arthritis.

A more recent study from Olmstead County in the USA reported that the survival in patients with psoriatic arthritis was not different from that of the general population. Since there have been advances in managing patients with psoriatic arthritis, a study which investigated whether mortality risk has changed over the last decade in the University of Toronto Psoriatic Arthritis Clinic was performed. This most recent study published in 2007 shows that while there still is an increased mortality risk, it has decreased over the past 2 decades. Currently the reduction in survival among patients with psoriatic arthritis followed in the Clinic compared with the Ontario population is only 3 years. This study suggests that the interventions in treating patients with psoriatic arthritis may have improved survival.

Quality of life in patients with psoriatic arthritis

Several studies within the University of Toronto Psoriatic Arthritis Clinic have demonstrated that patients with psoriatic arthritis have reduced quality of life compared with healthy controls. There are a number of questionnaires which have been developed to assess quality of life. Some of these are disease specific, while others are more generic. The generic instruments have an advantage in that they allow comparison of the disease with other diseases. While quality of life in patients with psoriatic arthritis is not totally related to the disease manifestations, these contribute about 50% to the quality of life. Results from clinical trials have also shown that new medications which work for skin and joint manifestations have improved the quality of life of the patients who used them.

Function in patients with psoriatic arthritis

A number of instruments have been developed to assess function in patients with psoriatic arthritis. The one most commonly used is the Health Assessment

Questionnaire (HAQ). Patients with psoriatic arthritis have reduced function compared with the general population. The reduced function is related partly to disease activity and partly to damage. Patients with more recent disease onset are able to improve their function much more than patients with longer disease duration. Therefore, patients should be identified and treated early in order to avoid permanent reduction in function as a result of the psoriatic arthritis.

Fatigue

Patients with psoriatic arthritis suffer from fatigue much more commonly than the general population. Two instruments to measure fatigue were validated in the University of Toronto Psoriatic Arthritis Program: the Fatigue Severity Scale (FSS) and the FACIT-fatigue scale. Both demonstrated that patients with psoriatic arthritis indeed suffer from fatigue, and their scores are different from those of the general population. Fatigue is associated with disease activity in patients with psoriatic arthritis. Several of the new agents used in psoriatic arthritis lead to a significant reduction in the fatigue scores in these patients.

Mechanisms of disease studies

Immunology

Studies from the University of Toronto Psoriatic Arthritis Clinic attempted to identify immunological abnormalities in this disease. Earlier studies revealed that patients with psoriatic arthritis, as well as patients with uncomplicated psoriasis, have impaired function of T suppressor cells, which are responsible for regulating the activity of other cells. Further studies supported the concept of an immunological imbalance in lymphocyte populations in patients with psoriasis and psoriatic arthritis compared with healthy controls. The same abnormalities, however, were detected in patients with psoriatic arthritis as in patients with uncomplicated psoriasis.

Genetics

Family investigations

Genetic factors are thought to be important in the development of both psoriasis and psoriatic arthritis. Forty per cent of the patients in the University of Toronto Psoriatic Arthritis Clinic reported a family history of a first-degree relative (parent, sibling, or child) having either psoriasis or psoriatic arthritis. Patients who report a family history of psoriatic arthritis have an earlier age of onset and present with less severe disease than patients who do not have a family history. It is likely that patients who have relatives with the disease are more alert to the symptoms of joint disease and thus present immediately as opposed to waiting until the symptoms become very severe. There is an increased transmission of the disease through the father, a fact which is important when performing genome-wide scans.

At the University of Toronto Psoriatic Arthritis Clinic, patients who agree to their family members being contacted participate in family investigations. All available relatives of patients with psoriatic arthritis are evaluated clinically with a standard protocol which is a shortened version of the usual Clinic protocol. Where indicated, that is when it is suspected that a person may have some form of arthritis, the relatives undergo X-ray assessment. An initial study compared the patient's ability to identify the presence of either psoriasis or psoriatic arthritis in their relatives with the findings at clinical examination. The results showed that while patients were pretty accurate at identifying relatives with psoriasis, they were only 50% correct in identifying relatives with psoriatic arthritis. For that reason it was important to evaluate all relatives for the purpose of psoriatic arthritis.

A recent study was undertaken to determine the risk of psoriasis and psoriatic arthritis among family members of patients with psoriatic arthritis. One hundred consecutive families were collected and 287 first-degree relatives participated in the study. It was determined that 7.6% of the relatives had psoriatic arthritis while 15.3% had psoriasis. Based on a prevalence of psoriatic arthritis of 0.25% and of psoriasis of 2%, the risk ratio for psoriatic arthritis was calculated at 30.4 while that for psoriasis was calculated at 7.6. These numbers clearly demonstrate a significant familial predisposition to psoriasis and psoriatic arthritis.

Identifying susceptibility genes for psoriasis and psoriatic arthritis

Specific studies to identify the genes involved in the susceptibility to psoriasis and psoriatic arthritis began with HLA studies in the mid-1980s. HLA is the major histocompatibility complex of man located on the short arm of chromosome 6p. This area was originally discovered in relation to the transplantation programme when it was noted that organs transplanted in certain individuals would be rejected while in others they were not. It turned out that similarities in the HLA system allowed transplants to be accepted, while differences led to transplant rejection. The HLA region was subsequently found to be important in various immune functions. HLA was also found to be an important area in susceptibility to immune-mediated diseases. The first HLA study from the University of Toronto Psoriatic Arthritis Clinic was published in 1984.

The study included 158 patients with psoriatic arthritis and 101 patients with psoriasis who did not have arthritis. Both groups were compared with healthy controls. There was an increased frequency of certain HLA antigens in both psoriasis and psoriatic arthritis compared with controls. The main differences between patients with psoriatic arthritis and those with uncomplicated psoriasis were the increased frequency of HLA-B7 and HLA-B27 among patients with psoriatic arthritis, and the increased frequency of HLA-Cw6 and HLA-DR7 in patients with psoriasis without arthritis. These studies supported the genetic predisposition to psoriasis and psoriatic arthritis, and suggested that there may be genetic differences in the predisposition to psoriatic arthritis and uncomplicated psoriasis. We also found that certain HLA antigens were associated with less severe disease, while others were associated with disease progression. Further studies demonstrated that HLA-Cw6 was associated with an earlier age of onset of psoriasis among patients with psoriatic arthritis.

Another family study, this time looking at siblings (brothers and sisters) of patients with psoriatic arthritis, was also performed at the University of Toronto Psoriatic Arthritis Clinic. The siblings who had psoriatic arthritis were compared with the siblings who only had psoriasis or were not affected at all by either psoriasis or arthritis. There was an increase in haplotype sharing (sharing of identical segments of genes) among siblings concordant for psoriatic arthritis compared with those who were unaffected or who had psoriasis. This provided additional support for the familial predisposition and for the role of HLA in the susceptibility to psoriatic arthritis.

Other susceptibility genes

Another approach to identifying genetic factors for susceptibility to psoriasis and psoriatic arthritis is a genome-wide scan. This method involves either family studies for linkage, or association studies where cases are compared with controls. Unfortunately, these methods are very expensive and we have not yet been able to garner the funds to support such an effort. However, we have been able to perform association studies with candidate genes. These are genes which are thought to be important based on other studies. For example, we know that the HLA region is important. We also know that certain genes in that region are important. We have therefore concentrated on genes within the HLA region and performed studies using single nucleotide polymorphisms, or SNPs. These are variations in a single nucleotide which lead to different proteins and may thus be important not only as markers but sometimes in specific protein expression. We have found that there is a **tumour necrosis factor-**α (TNF-α) polymorphism associated with psoriatic arthritis. We have also found that certain SNPs previously shown to be associated with psoriasis were not associated with psoriatic arthritis. In a novel approach, we pooled DNA from 250 patients and compared it with that of 250 controls, and we found a new area to be associated with psoriatic arthritis. Other candidate genes found to be associated with psoriatic arthritis include the interleukin-1 (IL-1) gene on chromosome 1 and IL-23 gene on chromosome 2.

However, we still aim to perform the definitive analysis of a genome-wide scan. To do this we have joined forces with other investigators so that we can have a large enough sample and raise the funds to perform the study.

Treatment

Traditional disease-modifying medications

The University of Toronto Psoriatic Arthritis Clinic provided an opportunity to investigate the effectiveness of treatment used in psoriatic arthritis. Two approaches have been taken: one in which we analysed the effect of therapy on the patients followed longitudinally using the database, and the other through participating in randomized controlled trials.

Initial efforts investigated the traditional medications used for the treatment of psoriatic arthritis. The first study tested whether gold therapy was able to prevent progression of joint damage in psoriatic arthritis, and proved that it did not. The effectiveness of chloroquine, an antimalarial which had been considered bad for patients with psoriasis as it was thought to aggravate the psoriasis, was tested next. It was found that chloroquine may work for some patients, and that it clearly did not worsen the psoriasis. However, to prove the efficacy, a much larger study would be required.

Methotrexate has long been considered a useful drug in psoriasis and psoriatic arthritis. Interestingly, though, there are no good randomized controlled trials which demonstrate its efficacy in either skin or joint disease. Nonetheless, studies have shown that in practice most dermatologists and rheumatologists think it works very well and use it frequently. The study based on the University of Toronto Psoriatic Arthritis Clinic database showed that methotrexate did not prevent progression of joint damage in patients with psoriatic arthritis. There was some criticism of the study in that although it was case-controlled, it included a small number of patients, whose disease duration was long, and the dose of methotrexate may not have been high enough. In a recent survey of our Clinic, we found that we are now using methotrexate earlier in the course before there is a lot of damage, and it may actually work better under these circumstances. However, despite the fact that the inflammation appears to be better controlled with higher doses of methotrexate, we still do not have any evidence that methotrexate actually prevents progression of joint damage.

The effectiveness of azathioprine in psoriatic arthritis was tested next. There are no controlled studies with this drug, but case series have suggested that it works. Azathioprine was found to work for both skin and joints in some patients, but it too did not prevent progression of joint damage.

Sulfasalazine is a medication that was specifically developed for rheumatoid arthritis. In early studies it did not seem to work very well and it was then tested in inflammatory bowel disease and was found to work well. In the past 20 years there have been several randomized controlled trials of sulfasalazine in patients with psoriatic arthritis. It provides marginal benefit over placebo with regards to joint inflammation. The study based on the University of Toronto Psoriatic Arthritis Clinic database demonstrated that a large proportion of the patients could not take the drug because of side effects and, in those who continued to take it, there was no protection from progression of joint damage.

Patients attending the University of Toronto Psoriatic Arthritis Clinic have participated in a number of randomized controlled trials. They tried leflunomide, a medication similar to methotrexate, as part of the TOPAS trial. The trial showed a modest effect of leflunomide on the inflammatory process, but unfortunately the drug was not tested for its effect on prevention of damage. While the drug may work well in about 40% of the patients, it is either not tolerated or ineffective in the remainder of the patients.

Biological therapies for psoriatic arthritis

The most exciting discovery for patients with psoriasis and psoriatic arthritis has been the development of the biological agents. Among them, the anti-TNF agents have been the most successful. Three drugs, etanercept, infliximab, and adalimumab, have shown a remarkable improvement in signs and symptoms of skin and joint manifestations. These drugs also work to improve quality of life and function, and, importantly, they prevent the progression of joint damage. Indeed, for both infliximab and adalimumab, it has been shown that the drug can overcome the predictive effect of CRP in progression of joint damage. At the University of Toronto Psoriatic Arthritis Clinic we were able to show that etanercept works well among our patients with psoriatic arthritis and is very well tolerated. We also participated in the infliximab trials as well as the adalimumab trials, both of which provided excellent response. The experience in our Clinic with these drugs has been very rewarding.

On the other hand, other biological agents approved for psoriasis, including efalizumab and alefacept, both T cell agents, have not worked well for psoriatic arthritis. Efalizumab may actually aggravate arthritis, while the effect of alefacept, which was studied only in conjunction with methotrexate, was quite modest. Neither drug was studied for the effect on joint damage progression.

Thus, patients with psoriatic arthritis now have several options to control both skin and joint manifestations which also prevent progression of joint damage. The difficulty is that these medications are very expensive and are not available for all patients. Those who have drug coverage through private health insurance or through government programmes must have at least five swollen joints and must have tried both methotrexate and leflunomide before the anti-TNF agents can be provided for them. The psoriasis must be very severe before any biological agent is provided on the basis of psoriasis. It is hoped that with time the cost of these drugs will go down and they will become more readily available. The information gathered through the University of Toronto Psoriatic Arthritis Program indicates that if patients are treated more appropriately earlier in the course of their disease they may not progress and may survive longer. It is possible that if patients are provided with these drugs that work more efficiently they may not need to take them for prolonged periods, and in the long run it will be much more cost effective.

Current and future studies

The University of Toronto Psoriatic Arthritis Program continues to evaluate the course and outcome in patients with psoriatic arthritis. The direct relationship between inflammation and damage in an individual joint is currently under investigation. We are also looking at the relationship between control of inflammation and prevention of joint damage. We are collaborating with colleagues worldwide to try and identify the genes responsible for the development of psoriatic arthritis in patients with psoriasis. To that end, we are also looking to identify the psoriatic arthritis early to determine whether we can change the course of the disease by instituting drugs earlier. We are interested in the relationship between genetic factors and response to treatment, as well as development of adverse reactions to drugs. We continue to develop protocols for new drug trials and participate in the trials, and we hope that our genetic studies will identify new targets for therapeutic interventions.

Summary

So what are the lessons learnt from the University of Toronto Psoriatic Arthritis Program?

- The first lesson is that a longitudinal observational cohort which is well characterized provides a unique opportunity to study a disease. As long as one is as careful about the details in a clinical observational cohort as in a randomized controlled trial or in a laboratory study, the science can be excellent.

- The University of Toronto Psoriatic Arthritis Program has helped understand the clinical course of psoriatic arthritis. It proved that the disease was more severe than previously thought and that inflammation leads to damage and early mortality. Those are modifiable factors and with the right approaches can be offset.

- We have learnt that the drugs traditionally used for psoriatic arthritis have not modified the course of the disease, but that new drugs work much better.

- We have identified some of the genetic and immunological factors which are responsible for developing psoriasis and psoriatic arthritis, but these still need further refinement.

14

International collaborations

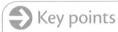 Key points

- Psoriatic arthritis is a complex disease

- In order to study the various aspects of the disease, international collaboration between rheumatologists, dermatologists, and other investigators is necessary

- The Group for Research and Assessment of Psoriasis and Psoriatic Arthritis (GRAPPA) was developed to facilitate international collaborations

- Through GRAPPA, a number of international collaborations have developed, beginning with evaluation of treatment modalities and treatment recommendations

- It is hoped that through these efforts the cause and mechanism of psoriasis and psoriatic arthritis will be identified, and better treatments will be developed

The first description of psoriatic arthritis is attributed to a French physician, Dr Alberti, who described the arthritis associated with psoriasis. However, in 1939, a prominent American rheumatologist, Dr Bauer, claimed that there was not enough in the description of the arthritis associated with psoriasis to distinguish it as a unique entity. Subsequent studies led to the recognition of psoriatic arthritis as a unique entity in the 1950s. Psoriatic arthritis was finally recognized as a unique form of arthritis by the American Rheumatism Association (now known as the American College of Rheumatology) in 1964.

Investigations into psoriatic arthritis

Psoriatic arthritis was originally thought of as a rare, mild disease, and therefore there was not a great interest in studying it among investigators. It was the late Professor Verna Wright of Leeds, UK who raised awareness of psoriatic arthritis in the late 1950s. He is therefore credited with recognizing psoriatic arthritis as a unique entity, and with the description of its varied clinical patterns. Several individuals have worked on the disease between the 1950s and the late 1990s. The majority of investigators working on psoriatic arthritis were in Europe. Several groups in the UK, Spain, and Italy have worked on this condition for the past three decades. In North America, the study of psoriatic arthritis was limited to a few groups, a group in Toronto, Canada, and two groups in the USA. While each of these groups was working alone, the studies published from the different centres by and large confirmed each other's findings. Initial studies concentrated on the clinical picture of psoriatic arthritis, with subsequent studies investigating the mechanisms of disease in terms of both genetics and immunology, as well as pathology of the lesions of both the skin and the joints.

Understanding psoriatic arthritis at the turn of the twenty-first century

Based on the investigations carried out in patients with psoriatic arthritis over the past 20 years, it has become apparent that the disease was not as rare as previously thought, and that it was much more severe. It was demonstrated that patients with psoriatic arthritis may develop a very severe, destructive form of arthritis that leads to marked disability. Several studies confirmed that genetic factors were important in the development of psoriatic arthritis, and that certain immunological abnormalities were associated with the disease. While the pathological appearance of psoriatic arthritis resembled that of rheumatoid arthritis, certain differences were observed, suggesting that different mechanisms may be responsible for these different forms of inflammatory arthritis. That background, together with the availability of biological agents which were shown to be effective for psoriasis and psoriatic arthritis since 2000, has led to a greater interest in identifying the cause and the exact mechanisms of this form of arthritis, and its relationship to psoriasis.

The exact frequency of the occurrence of psoriatic arthritis is unknown. However, it is possible that it is as frequent as rheumatoid arthritis, which is the typical form of inflammatory arthritis. An individual physician in a primary care setting may encounter only a few patients with psoriatic arthritis. A specialist rheumatologist or dermatologist will probably encounter many more patients with psoriatic arthritis. However, in order to understand the disease better, it is necessary to study large numbers of patients, particularly when studies involve identifying genes associated with the disease or its severity. Since none of the groups has had enough patients on its own, it was necessary to build collaborations among investigators, in order to increase the number of subjects studied, and to enlarge the scope of the study. In addition, as more individuals became interested in the disease, it became clear that education of health care professionals, patients, and the public at large was necessary to allow earlier diagnosis and treatment of individuals suffering from psoriatic arthritis.

Historically, dermatologists were working on identifying the causes and the mechanisms associated with the psoriatic skin disease, and by and large ignored the presence of arthritis. While the presence of arthritis denoted more severe disease in patients with psoriasis, the dermatologists did not pay close attention to whether their patients actually suffered from arthritis unless the patient complained of it specifically. Rheumatologists on the other hand have concentrated on the peripheral arthritis, the back involvement, as well as the associated features of dactylitis (swollen digits known as sausage digits) and enthesitis (inflammation at the insertion of tendons into bone), and have not paid close attention to the skin disease. Thus, many patients with inflammatory arthritis may be misdiagnosed as having rheumatoid arthritis since the psoriasis was not identified by the primary care physician or the rheumatologist. In many centres, dermatologists and rheumatologists work totally independently and it is difficult to obtain a consultation from one or the other. Some centres have rheumatologists and no dermatologists, and others have dermatologists and no rheumatologists. Only recently has it become clear that a team approach to this disease is preferred.

Better recognition of psoriatic arthritis—the beginnings of international collaboration

The definition of psoriatic arthritis that was used until recently has not been precise. Although most investigators and clinicians used the clinical description of Moll and Wright published in the early 1970s as diagnostic criteria, these described clinical patterns but were not necessarily helpful in early disease. Until 2006 there had not been a widely accepted and valid classification or diagnostic criteria for psoriatic arthritis. To address this problem, an international group of investigators got together under the leadership of Drs Philip Helliwell of Leeds, UK, and William Taylor of Wellington, New Zealand. They gathered a group of 30 investigators from 17 countries worldwide. Through the efforts of this group which became known as CASPAR

(ClASsification of Psoriatic ARthritis), a large number of patients and controls were evaluated according to a standard protocol. From the information gathered in that study, classification criteria were derived through statistical methods. These criteria proved very sensitive (able to pick up cases with psoriatic arthritis) and specific (able to distinguish patients with psoriatic arthritis from those with other forms of inflammatory arthritis) for the diagnosis of psoriatic arthritis. These are called the CASPAR criteria. The CASPAR criteria will be used to identify patients for clinical trials and longitudinal studies of patients with psoriatic arthritis. These criteria are useful in established psoriatic arthritis, in early psoriatic arthritis, and even in a family medicine clinic to assist physicians in arriving at the correct diagnosis.

The Group for Research and Assessment of Psoriasis and Psoriatic Arthritis

From the initial gathering of the CASPAR group arose another idea to assemble individuals interested in the study of psoriatic arthritis internationally. This effort was organized by Drs Philip Mease of Seattle, USA, and Dafna Gladman of Toronto, Canada. The aim was to get together rheumatologists and dermatologists as well as other investigators interested in psoriasis and psoriatic arthritis. The initial plan was to gather together at a workshop as many such individuals as possible from various centres around the world, to provide an opportunity to review current knowledge, identify gaps in current knowledge, and propose new avenues for research in this condition. In particular, the purpose was to bring together individuals from different disciplines such that there would be 'cross-fertilization'. The group convened for the first time in New York in August 2003. Despite the fact that there was a blackout on the Eastern seaboard of the USA that weekend, a fact which restricted the arrival of several of the intended participants, the meeting went ahead successfully and led to the establishment of the Group for Research and Assessment of Psoriasis and Psoriatic Arthritis (GRAPPA).

GRAPPA is an international group of rheumatologists, dermatologists, and methodologists committed to achieving the following goals:

- Increase awareness and early diagnosis of psoriasis and psoriatic arthritis

- Develop and validate assessment tools

- Evaluate treatment modalities in order to promote clinical research with the ultimate goal of improving disease outcome

- Promote basic research into disease pathophysiology

◆ Foster interdisciplinary communication

◆ Foster communication with the general public via patient service leagues, industry, regulatory agencies, and other concerned bodies.

GRAPPA members have been meeting to review their work and develop new research efforts on a regular basis. Meetings usually occur adjacent to rheumatology meetings such as the American College of Rheumatology in North America, and the EUropean League Against Rheumatism (EULAR) meeting in Europe, as well as adjacent to dermatology meetings such as the American Academy of Rheumatology (AAD) in North America and the European Academy of Dermatology and Venereology (EADV) in Europe. While these are important meetings, the participation is usually limited to specialists attending meetings pertaining to their specialties, thus there is less interaction between rheumatologists and dermatologists. Nonetheless, several topics have been discussed and agreed upon.

Since 2003, members of GRAPPA have worked tirelessly to achieve the goals of the group. Over the past 4 years there has been a steady increase in the number of abstracts accepted to national and international meetings on psoriasis and psoriatic arthritis. This raises the awareness about this disease among rheumatologists and dermatologists. Moreover, the proceedings of the 2003 inaugural meeting of GRAPPA have been published as a supplement to the *Annals of the Rheumatic Diseases*, the official journal of EULAR. These proceedings are available on the Internet as a free service through an arrangement between the *Annals* and GRAPPA. This publication has also raised awareness about the disease. More specialist physicians are now trying to arrive at an earlier diagnosis. However, we still have work to do in terms of primary care physicians referring patients to the appropriate specialist so that the diagnosis is made as early as possible. We also must make sure that public awareness is heightened so that patients seek medical attention in a timely manner.

Assessment tools in psoriatic arthritis—GRAPPA collaborations

GRAPPA members have been involved in the development and validation of assessment tools for psoriasis and psoriatic arthritis. Because psoriatic arthritis has peripheral joint manifestations (affecting the joints of the extremities) as well as the joints of the spine, and affecting the skin and nails, there are several aspects of the disease that require assessment. GRAPPA began this process at its initial meeting in 2003 and continued it through links with other international groups, including the Outcome Measures in Rheumatology Clinical Trials (OMERACT), the Ankylosing Spondylitis Assessment (ASAS) group, the SPondyloArthritis

Research Consortium Canada (SPARCC), the SPondyloARthritis Treatment Assessment Network (SPARTAN), and the International Psoriasis Council (IPC). Through these efforts, a consensus on a core set of domains to be included in clinical trials and observational cohort studies in psoriatic arthritis has been achieved. The instruments necessary for the areas of assessment (called domains) have either been validated already, or are currently undergoing validation through GRAPPA participating centres. Papers describing these instruments and their validation have been published, and it is hoped that physicians worldwide will be using these methods to assess their patients.

GRAPPA treatment recommendations

A major effort of GRAPPA has been the development of internationally agreed upon treatment recommendations for psoriasis and psoriatic arthritis. This was achieved through a critical review of the literature of the treatment modalities currently used for both skin and joint manifestations. The review was published in the *Journal of Rheumatology* in 2006, and provides the cornerstone for the recommendations which will be published within the next few months. This is the result of a tireless effort of the Treatment Guidelines Committee of GRAPPA, co-chaired by Christopher Ritchlin of Rochester, New York, and Arthur Kavanaugh of San Diego, California, with help from several GRAPPA members, both dermatologists and rheumatologists, who served on the committee, as well as the membership at large who participated in discussions and surveys to arrive at a common resolution.

Current membership of GRAPPA includes rheumatologists, dermatologists, radiologists, methodologists, nurses, and other health professionals, members of patient groups such as the National Psoriasis Foundation in the USA and members of the International Federation of Psoriasis Associations (IFPA), as well as pharmaceutical representatives. At present, the majority are from outside North America.

International world congress on psoriasis and psoriatic arthritis

In 2006 the first world congress on psoriasis and psoriatic arthritis was held in Stockholm, Sweden. The Congress was the brainchild of the executive of IFPA. Under the leadership of Drs Mark Lebwohl of New York, Kenneth Gordon of Chicago, and Philip Mease of Seattle, and with the help of the research director of the National Psoriasis Foundation of the USA, a steering committee which included Dafna Gladman (Toronto, Canada), Christopher Ritchlin (Rochester, New York, USA), and Mona Stahle (Stockholm, Sweden), and a scientific committee which included international representation of both rheumatologists and dermatologists, an outstanding scientific programme was put together. More than 700 people attended the meeting which included four themes: genetics, immunology, quality of life and burden of disease, and clinical research. Each section was co-chaired by a rheumatologist and dermatologist, with contributions to the session by both disciplines. There were review lectures and original research presentations in each of the sections. There were also poster sessions related to each of these themes. After each section there was a summary session for the patients which provided information in lay terms. At the end of the meeting there was a patient advocacy meeting which provided an opportunity for discussion of issues affecting patients with psoriasis and psoriatic arthritis around the world. The success of the meeting is most probably due to the commitment and hard work of the executive directors of IFPA. Proceedings of the meeting were published in the *Journal of Investigative Dermatology*.

This was the first opportunity for many rheumatologists and dermatologists to meet together to discuss issues related to psoriasis and its associated arthritis. It was most productive to have researchers working on the genetics of psoriasis interacting with those working on the genetics of psoriatic arthritis. Likewise, dermatologists working on the immunology of skin psoriasis were able to identify common grounds for study with rheumatologists working on the immunology of joint disease. It became clear that quality of life and burden of disease issues affecting patients with psoriasis were even greater in those also suffering from arthritis. It also became clear that many associated diseases affecting patients with psoriatic arthritis, such as heart disease, obesity, and diabetes, were also affecting patients with psoriasis who did not have arthritis. The meeting surpassed the organizers' expectations, and there are already plans for the next meeting to be held in Stockholm in 2009.

Moving forward in the investigation of psoriatic arthritis

Most recently GRAPPA held its annual meeting in Boston, USA, in September 2007. This was another opportunity for rheumatologists, dermatologists, and basic scientists to get together to discuss common issues. This meeting included several components. A session on screening and assessment tools was co-chaired by Philip Mease of Seattle and Abrar Qureshi of Boston. Reviews of the instruments developed for the assessment of skin and joint manifestations were reviewed, and a research agenda was developed through breakout groups. A session on quality measures was co-chaired by Henning-Wulf Boehncke of Frankfurt, Germany, and Arthur Kavanaugh of San Diego, California, USA, to consider the requirements for physician assessment of patients with psoriasis and psoriatic arthritis. A broad session on translational research chaired by Christopher Ritchlin of Rochester, New York, USA, included three parts: a biomarker session chaired by Oliver FitzGerald of Dublin, Ireland; a genetics session co-chaired by Proton Rahman of St. John's, Newfoundland, Canada, and James T. Elder of Ann Arbor, Michigan, USA; and an imaging session co-chaired by Philip Helliwell of Leeds, UK, and Alice Gottlieb of Boston, USA. Updates on the research in each of these areas were presented, and subsequent meetings will further delineate the research agenda. At a session on drug therapy and toxicity co-chaired by Peter Nash of Australia and Alice Gottlieb of the USA, a review of data on methotrexate was presented as well as results of a survey of the use of methotrexate by rheumatologists and dermatologists. At a breakout group, plans for further studies and drug evaluations were made. The final session centred on registries and was co-chaired by Dafna Gladman of Toronto, Canada, and Mona Stahle of Stockholm, Sweden. The required content of clinical and genetic registries was discussed with the idea of developing an international registry for psoriasis and psoriatic arthritis.

An international collaborative effort to identify genes for psoriasis has been coordinated by James T. Elder, and has resulted in an important publication of the susceptibility genes in psoriasis. Further studies are required to identify genes for psoriatic arthritis, and whether these are different from those responsible for uncomplicated psoriasis.

Thus, the international collaborative efforts have helped the cause of patients with psoriasis and psoriatic arthritis. GRAPPA is planning to continue its work through annual meetings, as well as collaborative studies in between. A major international effort is centred on patient-related outcomes and the international classification of function which will further improve quality of life and function among patients with psoriasis and psoriatic arthritis. There are also plans to continue the world congresses every few years. Through these international collaborations, we hope that more studies will be performed and answers to many questions related to these conditions will be obtained. As a result, quality of life and function will improve, and one day the cause of and cure for both psoriasis and psoriatic arthritis will be identified.

Thus, these international collaborations have advanced our knowledge and understanding of disease mechanisms in psoriatic arthritis. They have also provided agreed-upon case definitions and assessment tools, and have incorporated patients' opinion into development of new tools. The expectation is that over the next few years the genetics of psoriatic arthritis will be understood and new therapeutic interventions be developed. It is also expected that these new drugs will be available to more individuals affected with the disease worldwide.

15

Current outlook for patients with psoriatic arthritis

 Key points

- The current situation for patients with psoriatic arthritis is much better than several years ago

- Research into the mechanism of the disease has led to the development of new therapeutic agents

- The new agents work much better than the older ones

- There is already evidence of improved survival in the past decade compared with the previous two decades

- The future is much brighter, with more drugs being developed and the opportunity to use the new drugs earlier in the course of the disease

- International groups serve an important role in ensuring that patients worldwide benefit from these new developments

The future for patients with psoriatic arthritis is shaping up to be much better than the past. Whereas at the beginning of the twentieth century the actual entity was not clear, towards the second half of the twentieth century the disease became recognized as a specific form of arthritis. Once this happened, more and more investigators began research into the nature, course, mechanism, and treatment of psoriatic arthritis.

The mechanism of inflammation is beginning to unravel

When one reviews the medical literature, one finds that there has been a tremendous increase in the number of publications related to psoriatic arthritis in all these areas of research. Indeed, extensive research into the mechanisms of the disease has been carried out recently. Some of this research, while not done specifically on psoriatic arthritis, is quite applicable. We have now recognized many of the molecules important in the development of inflammation which leads to the symptoms and signs of the disease. We also recognize that persistent inflammation leads to joint damage. The identification of the molecules responsible for inflammation has allowed the development of therapeutic agents which interfere with their ability to cause inflammation. Therefore, it may very well be that if we can turn off the inflammation early in the course of the disease, we will be able to prevent joint damage.

Improved survival in psoriatic arthritis over the past decade

Recent data from the University of Toronto Psoriatic Arthritis Program, which is the largest collection of patients with psoriatic arthritis followed prospectively, suggest that the survival has improved in the past decade. With the advent of successful treatment for psoriatic arthritis, with medications that not only control the signs and symptoms of inflammation but also prevent the progression of joint damage, the expectation is that there will be further improvement in the future.

Future therapies

Now that pharmaceutical companies are interested in developing drugs for psoriatic arthritis, it is expected that more effective and less toxic drugs will be developed. Hopefully, if these medications are provided in a timely fashion, before there is damage, then damage will be prevented altogether.

There are currently several drugs under investigation for psoriatic arthritis. Several of these drugs are in clinical trials, while others are still being investigated in laboratories around the world. Thus the disease process will eventually be conquered. It was recently recognized that patients with psoriatic arthritis are more susceptible to other medical problems such as heart attacks, diabetes, and high cholesterol. These clinical conditions are usually related to the 'burden of disease'. If the disease is controlled early in its course, its burden will be reduced and these complications should be avoided.

Availability of drugs

While the pharmaceutical companies are doing their best to develop and market new drugs for psoriatic arthritis, it should be noted that these new drugs are not readily available to all who would benefit from them. The new medications are very costly. It is clear that the pharmaceutical companies who developed these drugs have incurred major expenses in drug development, and should be reimbursed for these. However, the high cost of the drugs is prohibitive in developing countries. Even in the developed countries, not every individual is insured or is provided with the drug. Because of the high costs, several countries have developed guidelines for the use of these medications. Most require that other, cheaper drugs be used before an anti-TNF agent is allowed. While this may make sense financially, it may not make clinical sense, since we are trying to turn off the inflammation early, and it makes more sense to use drugs that work well early in the course. One problem that exists is that there are no clinical trials with these drugs in early psoriatic arthritis and there are no head to head comparisons with traditional drugs such as methotrexate. In the near future, we hope to carry out such studies that will convince both insurance companies and government agencies to provide these medications early in the course of the disease.

International efforts

The emergence of the Group for Research and Assessment of Psoriasis and Psoriatic Arthritis (GRAPPA) as well as efforts by the International Federation of Psoriasis Associations (IFPA) and national societies will probably result in further understanding of issues related to both psoriasis and psoriatic arthritis. GRAPPA is currently engaged in a number of collaborative studies looking at the mechanism of the disease, understanding patient-related issues, addressing assessment tools and quality improvement, and defining a state of minimal disease activity. These efforts will probably lead to better understanding of the disease as a whole. Because of their international stature, the results of these efforts will probably apply to patients with the disease worldwide.

The future

Based on the developments that took place within the last few years, the future is much brighter for patients with psoriatic arthritis. It is likely that within the next 5 years the genetic factors responsible for this disease will be elucidated. With the discovery of new genes, new opportunities for drug targets will be found. Researchers are working diligently to identify new molecules that are effective with minimal toxicity. There is, therefore, hope that over the next decade there will be great progress in this area such that the relatives of the current patients, who are at higher risk of developing the disease, may be identified and treated to prevent the disease from developing. All the while those who already have the disease will also benefit from the new therapies.

List of professional and patient advocacy organizations

Professional organizations

Group for Research and Assessment of Psoriasis and Psoriatic Arthritis (GRAPPA)
International Psoriasis Council (IPC)
American College of Rheumatology (ACR)
American Academy of Dermatology (AAD)
Canadian Rheumatology Association (CRA)
Canadian Dermatology Association (CDA)
Spondyloarthritis Research Consortium of Canada (SPARCC)
Spondyloarthritis Research and Treatment Network (SPARTAN)
The European League against Rheumatism (EuLAR)
European Academy of Dermatology and Venereology (EADV)
Indian Rheumatology Association (IRA)
Asia-Pacific League of Associations for Rheumatology (APLAR)
Pan-American League of Associations for Rheumatology (PANLAR)
The African League against Rheumatism (AFLAR)

Patient organizations

Psoriasis

Argentina

Name: Asociación Civil para el Enfermo de Psoriasis (AEPSO)
Contact: Silvia Fernandez Barrio
Address: Av. De Mayo 749-8 "48"
C1084AAP-Buenos Aires
Argentina
Tel: +54 11 43 42 1874/8328

Toll free: 0800 22 AEPSO (23776)
E-mail: info@aepso.org
Web site: www.aepso.org

Australia

Name: Psoriasis Australia Inc.
Contact: Helen McNair
Address: PO Box 290, Ashburton, VIC.
Australia 3147
Tel: +11 61 3 98138080
Fax: + 11 61 3 98138080
E-mail: pai@virtual.net.au
Web site: www.psoriasisaustralia.org.au

Belgium

Name: PSORIASIS LIGA VLAANDEREN vzw
Contact: Paul De Corte
Address: Beervelde-Dorp 39
9080 Lochristi
Belgium
Tel: +32 9 355 08 13
Fax: +32 9 355 08 13
E-mail: info@psoriasis-vl.be
Web site: www.psoriasis-vl.be

Canada

Name: Psoriasis Society of Canada
Contact: Judy Misner
Address: PO Box 25015
Halifax NS
Canada B3M 4H4
Tel: +1 902 443 8680
Fax: +1 902 443 2073
E-mail: judymisner@eastlink.ca
Web site: www.psoriasissociety.org

China

Name: China Psoriasis Foundation
Contact: Professor Yang Xue-Qin
Address: Department of Dermatology
Air Force General Hospital
30 Fucheng Road
Beijing 100036

PR China
Tel: +86 10 66928073
Fax: +86 10 6817 4056 or +86 10 669 28843
E-mail: Hy348829@hy.cgw.cn

Denmark

Name: Danmarks Psoriasis Forening
Contact: Karl Vilhelm Nielsen
Address: Kloverprisvej 10 B 1
DK-2650 Hvidovre
Denmark
Tel: +45 3675 5400
Fax: +45 3675 1403
E-mail: LK@psoriasis.dk
Web site: www.psoriasis.dk

Estonia

Name: Eesti Psoriaasiliit–EPsoL
Contact: Ms Tiina Põllumäge, Chairman
Address: Komeedi 13-4
10122 Tallinn
Estonia
Tel: +372 6 621 250
Fax: + 372 6 621 250
E-mail: Tiina.Pm@nlib.ee
Web site: www.epsol.ee

Finland

Name: The Finnish Psoriasis Association
Contact: Ingemo Törnroos
Address: Fredrikinkatu 27 A 3
FIN 00120 Helsinki
Finland
Tel: +358 9 2511 9011
Fax: +358 9 2511 9088
E-mail: ingemo.tornroos@psori.fi
Web site: www.psoriasisliitto.fi

France

Name: Association Pour la Lutte Contre le Psoriasis–APLCP
Contact: Patricia Jimmy/President Bernard Luet
Address: 68 Rue Romain Rolland
783 70 Plaisir

France
Tel: +33 1 30 54 72 60
E-mail: patricia.jimmy@ac-versailles.fr
Web site: www.aplcp.org

Germany

Name: Deutscher Psoriasis Bund e.V.
Contact: Professor Dr Joachim Barth
Address: Seewartenstraße 10
20459 Hamburg
Germany
Tel: +49 402233990
Fax: +49 4022339922
E-mail: jobarth@t-online.de
Web site: www.psoriasis-bund.de

Iceland

Name: Samtök Psoriasis og Exemsjúklinga (SPOEX)
Psoriasis and Eczema Association
Contact: Ms Valgerdur Audunsdottir
Address: Bolholti 6
105 Reykjavik
Iceland
Tel: +354 588 9666
Fax: +354 588 9622
E-mail: spoex@sporiasis.is
Web site: www.psoriasis.is

Indonesia

Name: Indonesian Psoriasis Care Foundation
(Yayasan Peduli Psoriasis Indonesia, YPPI)
Contact: Helena B Intan
Address: 23, Jl. Niaga Hijau 9
Jakarta 12310
Indonesia
Tel: +62 021 751 2614
Fax: +62 021 750 7739
E-mail: contact@psoriasisindonesia.org
Web site: www.psoriasisindonesia.org

Israel

Name: Israel Psoriasis Association
Contact: Dr Tamar Brosh
Address: 22 Derech Hashalom St.
Tel Aviv 67892
Israel
Tel: + 972 3 6247611
Fax: + 972 3 6247613
E-mail: psoriasis@bezeqint.net
Web site: www.psoriasis.org.il

Japan

Name: Japanese Psoriasis Association
Contact: Hitoshi Kobayashi, Head of Staff
Address: Hiraoka-Koen Higashi 3-choume, 9-3
Kiyota-ku, Sapporo, 004-0882
Japan
Tel: +81 11 738 5511
Fax: +81 11 739 5522
E-mail: hitoshi-kobayashi@hokkaido.med.or.jp
Web site: www.kansen-hkd.com

Kenya

Name: Psoriasis Association of Kenya
Contact: Dr Hoseah Waweru
Address: Upper Hill Medical Centre
5th Floor, Raph Bunche Road
PO Box 54802 00200 City Sq.
Nairobi
Kenya
Tel: +254 203 431 45
Fax: +254 20 343 143
E-mail: howaweru@skyweb.co.ke

Malta

Name: Psoriasis Association Malta
Contact: Ms Lucienne Tabone
Address: PO Box 2, Mosta
Malta
Tel: +356 21437606
E-mail: info@pam.org.mt
Web site: www.pam.org.mt

The Netherlands

Name: Psoriasis Vereniging Nederland
Contact: Mr A. Cats
Address: Diepenhorstlaan 2-H
2288 EW Rijswijk
The Netherlands
Tel: +31 703 836443
E-mail: secretariaat@pvnnet.nl
Web site: www.pvnnet.nl

New Zealand

Name: Psoriasis Association of New Zealand Inc.
Contact: Michael Oelsner (Pres)/Carolyn McGonnell (Sec)
Address: PO Box 44007
Lower Hutt
Wellington 5040
New Zealand
Tel: +64 4 5687 139/+64 4 569 4705
Fax: +64 4 5687 149/+64 4 569 4706
E-mail: psoriasis@xtra.co.nz

Norway

Name: Norwegian Psoriasis Association
Contact: Erik Nygaard
Address: PB 6547 Etterstad
0606 Oslo
Norway
Tel: +47 23 376240
Fax: +47 22 72 1659
E-mail: npf@psoriasis.no
Web site: www.psoriasis.no

Panama

Name: Psoriasis of Panama Foundation
Contact: Monica de Chapman
Address: Apartado Postal
0823-01628
Panamá
República de Panamá
Tel: +507 302 3855 or +507 302 3856
E-mail: informacion@psoriasispanama.org
Web site: www.psoriasispanama.org

Philippines

Name: Psorphil, Psoriasis Philippine Online Community Inc.
Contact: Josef de Guzman
Address: 2121-B, Luna Street,
Pasay City, Metro Manila
Philippines
Tel: +632 833 43 03
Fax: +632 833 43 03
E-mail: psoriasis.philippines@gmail.com
Web site: www.psorphil.org

Singapore

Name: The Psoriasis Association of Singapore
Contact: Dr Colin Theng (Pres) C/O National Skin Centre
Address: No 1 Mandalay Road
Singapore 308205
Tel: +65 63508551
E-mail: psoriasis_sg@yahoo.com
Web site: www.psoriasis.org.sg

South Africa

Name: South African Psoriasis Association
Contact: Catherine Alexander, Chairperson
Address: PO Box 801
Brackenfell 7561
South Africa
Tel: +27 21 556 1141 or +27 21 981 1650
Fax: +27 86 671 5009 or +27 21 981 1650
Cell +27 82 897 9854
E-mail: cathalex@sybaweb.co.za
Web site: www.sapsoriasis.co.za

Spain

Name: ACCIÓ PSORIASI
Contact: Juana Mª Del Molino
Address: HE Can Guardiola
C/. CUBA, 2
08030 Barcelona
Spain
Tel: +34 93 2804622
Fax: +34 93 2804280
E-mail: psoriasi@pangea.org
Web site: www.acciopsoriasi.org

Sweden

Name: Psoriasisförbundet, The Swedish Psoriasis Association
Contact: Annika Rastas
Address: Rökerigatan 19
121 62 Johanneshov
Sweden
Tel: +46 8 556 109 01
Fax: +46 8 556 109 19
E-mail: annika.rastas@pso.se
Web site: www.pso.se

Switzerland

Name: Schweizerische Psoriasis & Vitiligo Gesellschaft (SPVG)
Contact: Adelheid Witzeling, Secretary Office, Bern
Address: PO Box 1
3000 Bern 22
Switzerland
Tel: +41 31 359 90 99
Fax: +41 31 359 90 98
E-mail: info@spvg.ch
Web site: www.spvg.ch

Tanzania

Name: Psoriasis Association of Tanzania
Contact: Yassin Mgonda
E-mail: ymgonda@muchs.ac.tz

UK

Name: The Psoriasis and Psoriatic Arthritis Alliance/PAPAA
Contact: David and Julie Chandler, Directors
Address: PO Box 111
St Albans
Herts AL2 3JQ
UK
Tel: +44 8707703212
Fax: +44 870 7703213
E-mail: info@papaa.org
Web site: www.papaa.org
Scotland
Name: Psoriasis Scotland
Contact: Janice Johnson

Tel: +44 131 556 4117
E-mail: janice.johnson5@btinternet.com
Web site: www. psoriasisscotland.org.uk

USA

Name: National Psoriasis Foundation/USA
Contact: Gail Zimmerman, President & CEO
Address: 6600 SW 92nd Avenue, Suite 300
Portland, OR 97223
USA
Tel: + 1 503 244 7404
Fax: + 1 503 245 0626
E-mail: gzimmerman@psoriasis.org

Spondyloarthritis

Australia

Ankylosing Spondylitis Group of New South Wales
denisemckeon@bigpond.com
New South Wales
Ankylosing Spondylitis Group of Queensland
johnjohn@powerup.com.au
www.arthritis.org.au/asgroup
East Brisbane, Queensland
Ankylosing Spondylitis Group of Tasmania
mlimbric@tassie.net.au
Claremont, TAS 7011

Austria

Österreichische Vereinigung Morbus Bechterew (ÖVMB)
office@bechterew.at www.bechterew.at
Wien

Belgium

Vlaamse Vereniging voor Bechterew-patiënten v.z.w. (VVB) vvb@come.to
www.vvb.rheumanet.org
Knokke-Heist

Canada

Ankylosing Spondylitis Association of British Columbia (ASABC)
a-griddick@uniserve.com
Surrey, British Columbia

Manitoba Ankylosing Spondylitis Association +1 204 256 5320
Winnipeg, Manitoba
Ontario Spondylitis Association (OSA) info@spondylitis.ca
www.spondylitis.ca
Toronto, Ontario

Croatia

Croatian Ankylosing Spondylitis Society +385 1 37 87 248
Zagreb

Czech Republic

Klub Bechtereviku Klub.bechtereviku@seznam.cz www.sweb.cz/
Praha 2 klub.bechtereviku

Denmark

Gigtforeningen for Morbus Bechterew
torben@bechterew.dk www.bechterew.dk
København

France

Association Française des Spondylarthritiques (AFS)
afs@fr.st www.aplcp.org
Rennes

Germany

Deutsche Vereinigung Morbus Bechterew e.V. (DVMB)
dvmb@bechterew.de bechterew.de
Schweinfurt

Hungary

MEOSz Bechterew section +36 1 358 12 74
National Federation of Associations of Disabled Persons
Budapest

Ireland

Ankylosing Spondylitis Association of Ireland (ASAI)
info@ankylosing-spondylitis.ie
www.ankylosing-spondylitis.ie/
Dublin

Italy

Associazione Italiana Spondiloartriti (A.I.Sp.A) +39 0584 49083
Florence

Japan

Japan Ankylosing Spondylitis Club (JASC) +81 422 45 7985
Tokyo

Norway

Norsk Revmatikerforbund (NRF)/BEKHTEREV nrf.adm@rheuma.no
www.rheuma.no
Oslo

Portugal

Associação Nacional da Espondilite Anquilosante info@anea-sede.rcts.pt
www.anea.org.pt
(ANEA)

Singapore

Singapore Ankylosing Spondylitis Club (SASC) +65 6227-9726
www.arthritis.org.sg
Singapore

Slovenia

Drustvo za ankilozirajoci spondilitis Slovenije (DASS) dass@siol.net
Ljubljana

Switzerland

Schweizerische Vereinigung Morbus Bechterew (SVMB)
Société suisse de la spondylarthrite ankylosante (SSSA)
Societá svizzera morbo di Bechterew (SSMB) mail@bechterew.ch
www.bechterew.ch
Zürich

Taiwan

Ankylosing Spondylitis Caring Society of ROC wei3228@ms3.hinet.net
www.ascare.org.tw
Taipei

Turkey

Ankilozan Spondilit Hasta Dernegi (ASHAD) ashad@ashad.org
www.ashad.8m.comSpondylitis Association of America

UK

National Ankylosing Spondylitis Society (NASS) nass@nass.co.uk
www.nass.co.uk
Mayfield, East Sussex

Ukraine/Slovenia

Society of sufferers with Ankylosing Spondylitis
(Bechterew's Disease)
Fax +380 475 2172
Solotonosha
Ukraine

USA

Spondylitis Association of America (SAA) info@spondylitis.org
www.spondylitis.org
Sherman Oaks, CA

Glossary

Achilles tendon   Tendon at the back of the leg attaching the calf muscles to the heel bone

Actively inflamed joint count   A measure of the degree of joint inflammation in which the number of joints with swelling and/or tenderness is counted

Acute phase reactants   Proteins in the blood, the amount of which changes when systemic inflammation is present. Examples include C-reactive protein, erythrocyte sedimentation rate, and ferritin. These are used as a test for the presence of inflammation

Ankylosis   Joint destruction leading to complete fusion of the adjacent bones

Arthritis mutilans   A severe destructive form of psoriatic arthritis leading to shortening and destruction of fingers and toes. Arthritis mutilans is typical of psoriatic arthritis, but is fortunately uncommon

Arthroscope   An instrument used to visualize the inside of the joint. Minor procedures such as synovial biopsies and repair of damaged tissues can be done using an arthroscope

Asymmetric distribution   Distribution of arthritis in the extremities that does not involve the same joint on both sides of the body

Autoantibodies   Proteins produced by the immune system that attack the body's own antigens and cause destruction leading to autoimmune diseases

Autoimmune disease   Disease caused by primary dysfunction of the immune system in which immune cells and proteins attack organs in the body as though they are foreign. These diseases may be limited to an organ (e.g. Hashimoto's thyroiditis) or may affect multiple organs (e.g. systemic lupus erythematosus, rheumatoid arthritis)

Avascular necrosis of bone   A complication of steroid therapy where there is decreased blood supply to the bone especially in the hip joint, leading to destruction of bone and overlying cartilage

Complex genetic disease   Diseases in which environmental factors interact with genetic factors to cause disease. Most human diseases may be considered to be complex genetic diseases

Contractures   Deformities of joints where the joints are bent in a particular position and cannot straighten

Cytokines   Proteins produced by immune cells that mediate inflammation. TNF-α and interleukins are examples of cytokines

Dactylitis   Swelling of the whole digit, finger or toe. Results from inflammation in the joints and tendons, as well as the soft tissues

Demyelination   A condition in which there is loss of myelin, the covering on the nerves inside the brain and spinal cord, leading to loss of function of the affected nerves

Distal joints   End joints of the fingers and toes

Distal pattern   Pattern of psoriatic arthritis involving the end joints of the fingers or toes

Enthesitis   Inflammation at the insertion of tendons into bone

Epigenetic factors   Heritable factors that modify expression of genes depending on the parent of origin

Erythrocyte sedimentation rate   A blood test which reflects the degree of inflammation

Extra-articular   Involvement of body parts other than the joints

Flail joints   Joints which can be twisted every which way. This usually results from destruction of the joint, making it loose

Flexural psoriasis   A form of psoriasis occurring on the flexural areas such as under the arms, the groin, the anal cleft

Genetic association studies   Study design used to identify genes associated with a disease by comparing markers in a large number of patients and matched controls

Genetic linkage studies   Study design used to identify areas on chromosomes where genes responsible for a disease may be found using information from markers genotyped on a large number of families with members having the disease

Guttate psoriasis   A form of psoriasis with small skin lesions that look like tear drops

HLA antigens   Molecules on the surface of cells. The genes that code for these molecules reside on chromosome 6p in man

Immunosuppressants   Drugs that suppress the immune system and predispose to infection and sometimes cancer

Inflammatory bowel disease Disease characterized by abnormal inflammation of the lining of the intestines

Intra-articular injections Injections given into the joint usually in the clinic; may be given under ultrasound guidance

Iritis/uveitis Inflammation of the coloured structure in the eye surrounding the pupil

Ischaemic heart disease The most common type of heart disease due to narrowing of blood vessels from atherosclerosis

Joint fusion Or fused joints reflect the inability to move a joint in any direction. These usually result from bony bridging across the joint, termed ankylosis

Ligand A molecule on the cell surface which is necessary to connect with another molecule for immunologic activation or inhibition

Longitudinal observational cohort A type of study design in which a large number of subjects are observed over a prolonged duration, typically decades, to observe the varied clinical presentations, clinical course and outcome of a disease or condition

Macrophages A type of inflammatory cell seen in tissues, especially at sites of chronic inflammation

Multiple sclerosis A disease characterized by episodes of demyelination at various sites in the brain and spinal cord

Nail pitting Little holes in the nails which occur frequently among patients with psoriasis

Neutrophils A type of blood cell seen primarily at sites of early inflammation

Oligoarticular pattern A pattern of psoriatic arthritis where four or less joints are involved, usually not the same joints on both sides of the body

Onycholysis Separation of the nail from its bed

Osteoclasts Cells responsible for bone resorption and remodelling

Periostitis Inflammation of the periosteum, a thick membrane that covers bone. This often leads to separation of the membrane from bone and new bone formation

Peripheral joints Joints of the extremities

Placebo An agent used in drug trials which is inert pharmacologically and is used to compare the effect of the active agent being studied

Plantar fascia A tendon at the bottom of the foot inserting into the heel bone

Polyarticular pattern A pattern of psoriatic arthritis involving five or more joints

Psoriasis area and severity index (PASI)   A measure of the degree of skin inflammation which takes into account the average degree of redness, thickness, and scaling of psoriasis, and the body surface area affected by psoriasis

Psoriasis vulgaris   A red scaly rash which may occur in various parts of the body

Pustular psoriasis   A type of psoriasis with raised bumps on the skin filled with pus. This variety of psoriasis may involve only the palms and soles, or it may be more widespread

Rheumatoid factor   A protein which is present in the blood of over 85% of patients with rheumatoid arthritis and less than 15% of patients with psoriatic arthritis

Sacroiliac joint   The joint between the sacrum and the iliac bones at the back of the pelvis

Sacroiliitis   Inflammation of the sacroiliac joints

Seronegative   An individual who has a negative test for rheumatoid factor

Simple genetic diseases   Diseases caused by mutation in a gene coding for an important protein, usually causing a disease that is recognized in childhood. Examples include phenylketonuria, cystic fibrosis, and sickle cell disease

Spinal joints   Joints of the neck and back, and the sacroiliac joints of the pelvis

Spondylitis   Inflammation of the joints of the spine, including the neck, back, and sacroiliac joints

Spondylitis pattern   A pattern of psoriatic arthritis with the major manifestation being arthritis of the back (spinal) joints

Subcutaneous injection   An injection given into tissue under the skin, usually on the thigh or abdomen

Subluxation   A deformity in which the bones lose normal contact. There can be upward or downward subluxation where one bone moves above or below the other bone of the joint, or there can be sideways subluxation where one bone moves to one side or the other of the other bone

Subungual hyperkeratosis   Thickening of the nail bed

Syndesmophytes   Formation of bone in the outer layers of the discs between vertebrae

Synovectomy   Removal of the synovium. This can be done surgically or by injection of radioactive material into the joint

Synovial biopsies   Biopsy of the membrane lining the joint

Synovial fluid Fluid lubricating the joints. The amount and characteristics vary in different arthritic conditions, and its analysis helps in making the right diagnosis

Synovium Lining tissue of the joint

T cells A type of cell produced by the immune system that mediates the immune response towards various foreign antigens

Teratogenic Agents that cause harm to the foetus when given to pregnant women

Tumour necrosis factor (TNF) A factor produced by immune cells that is responsible for inflammation

Urethritis Inflammation of the urethra, the tube that lets urine out of the body from the bladder

Index